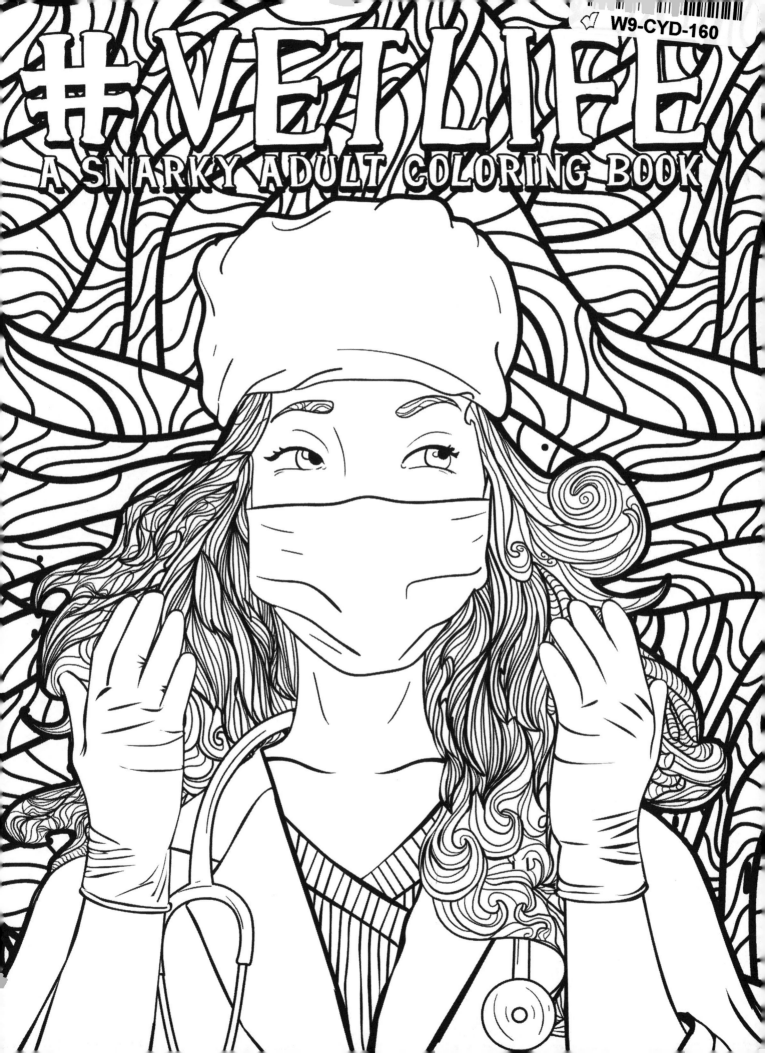

#VETLIFE
A SNARKY ADULT COLORING BOOK

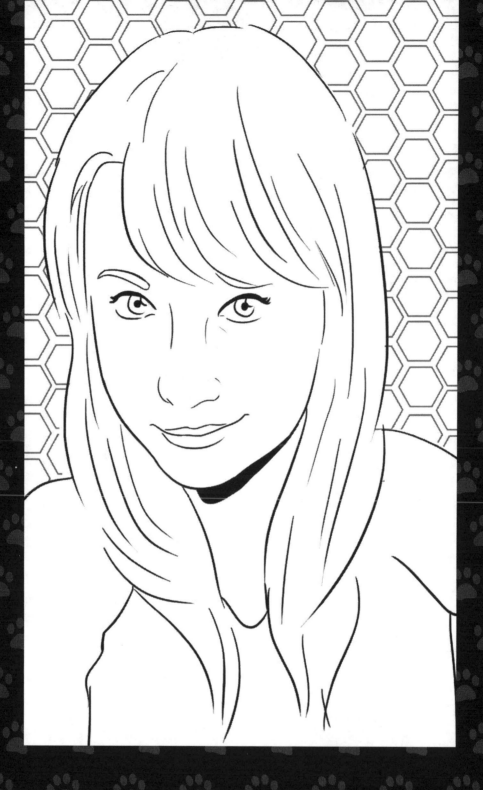

Illustrated by Micaela

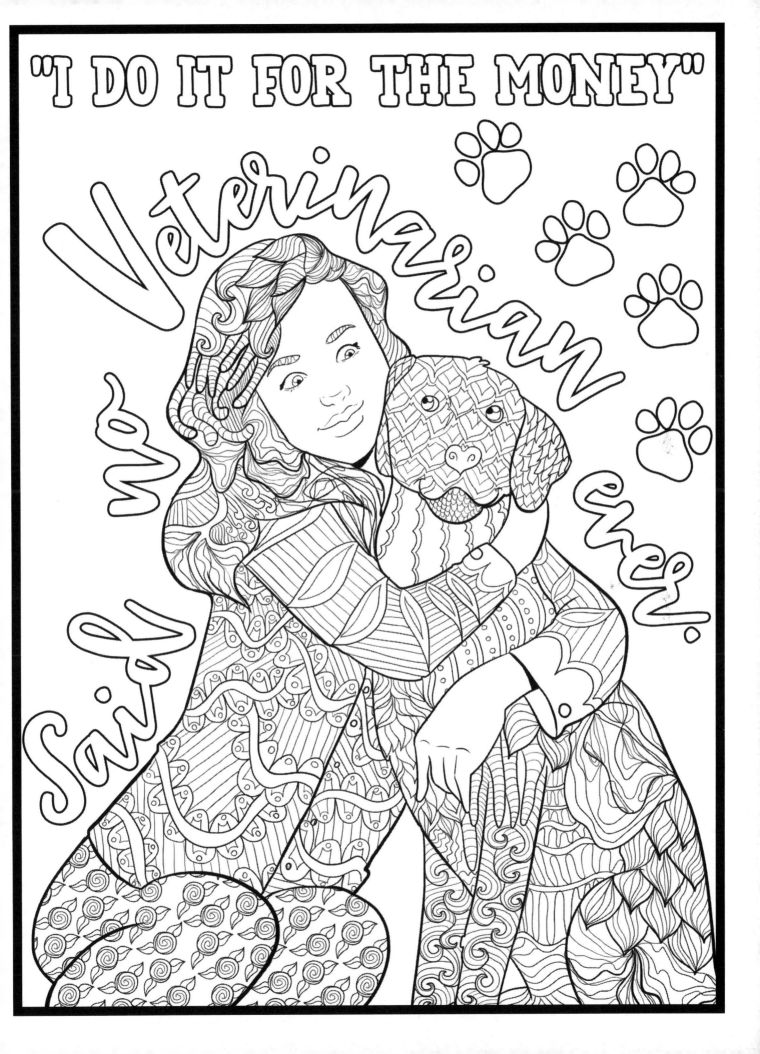

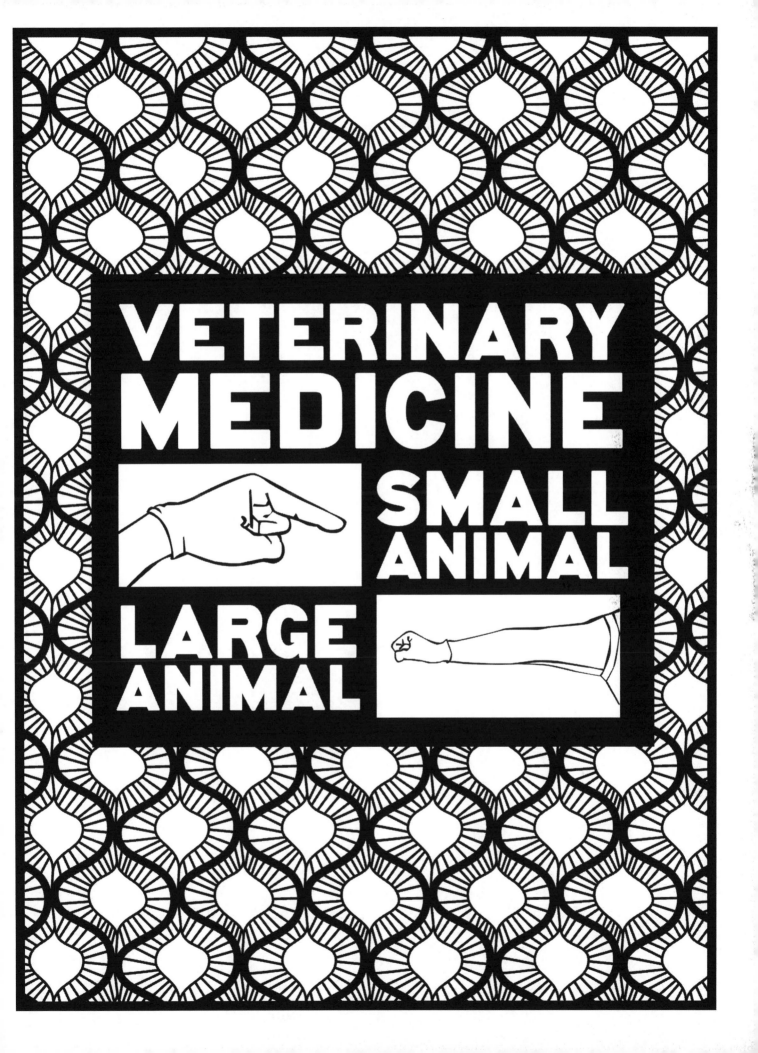

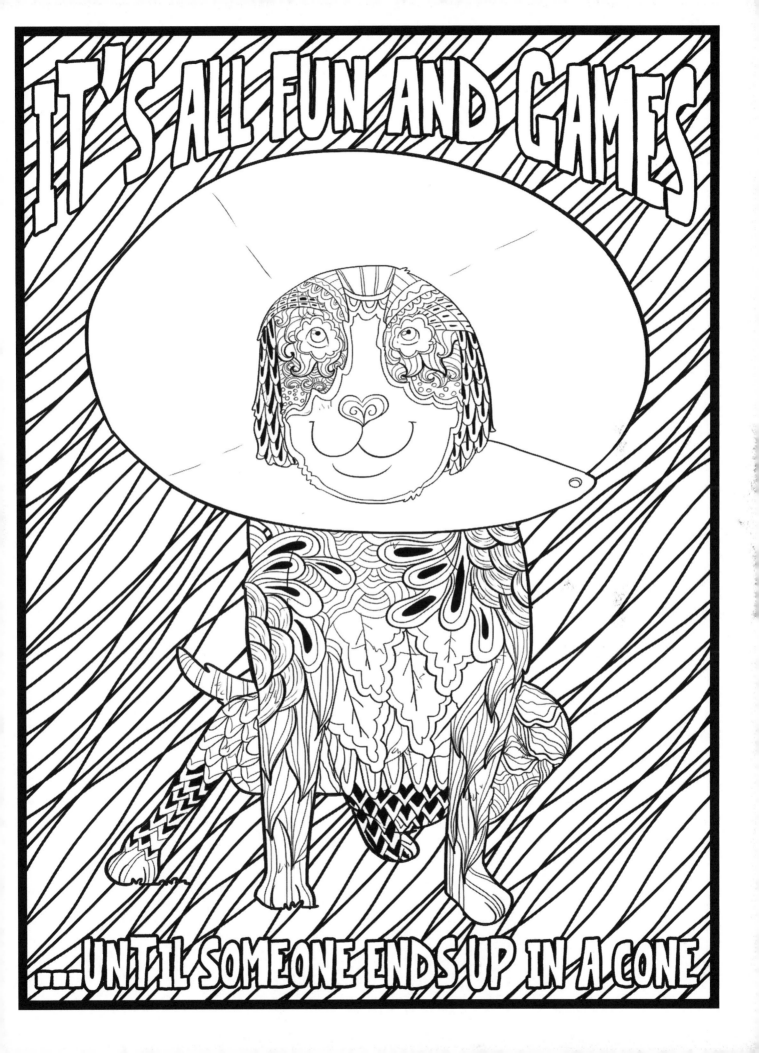

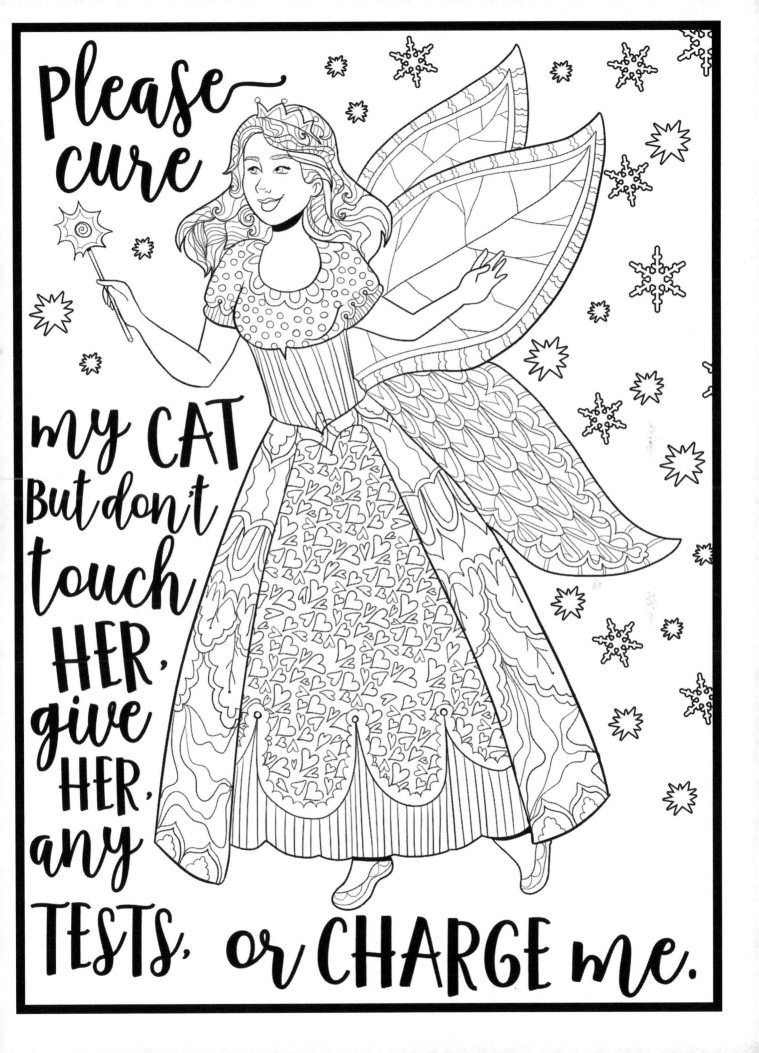

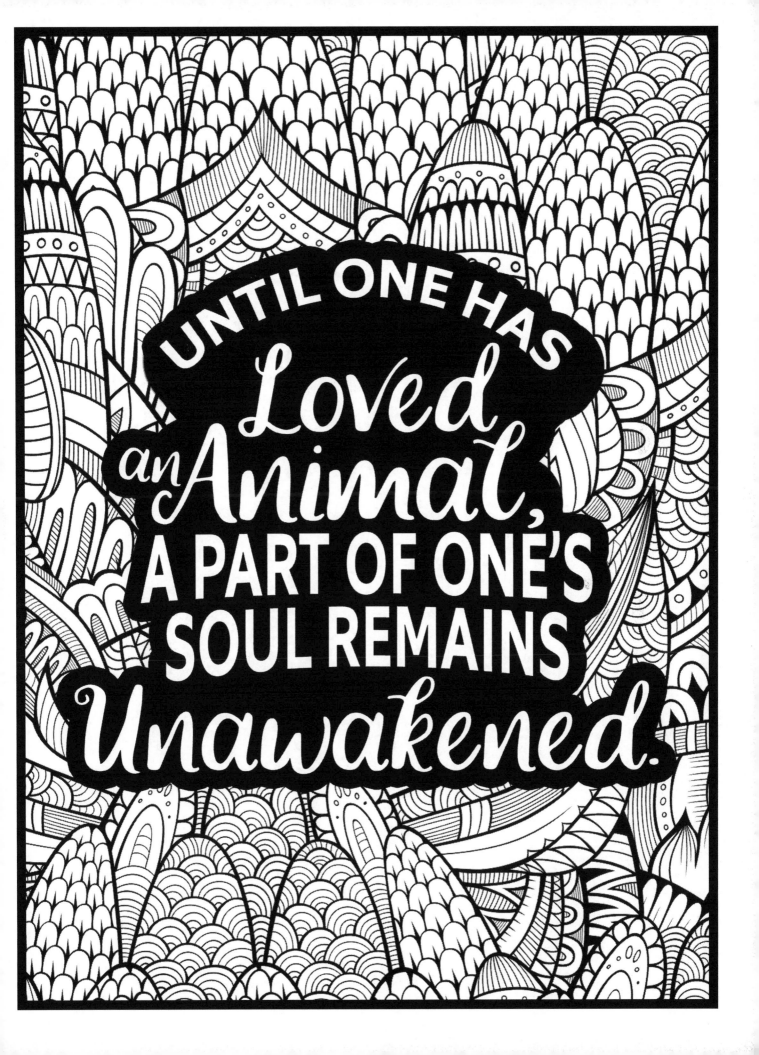

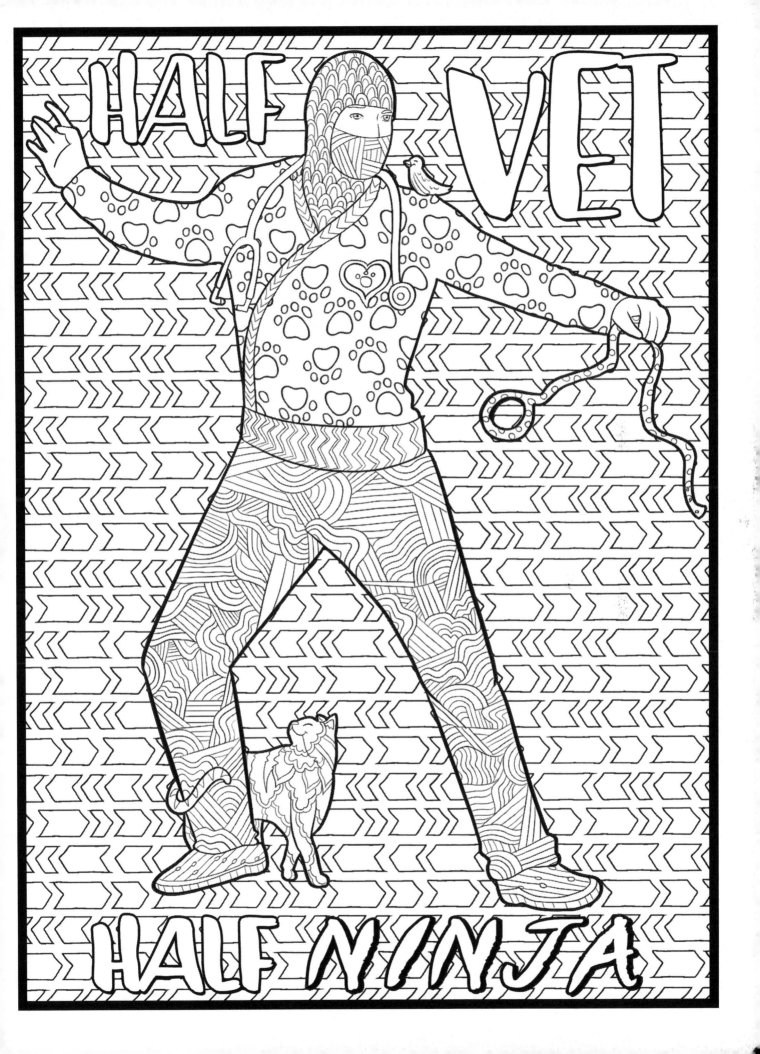

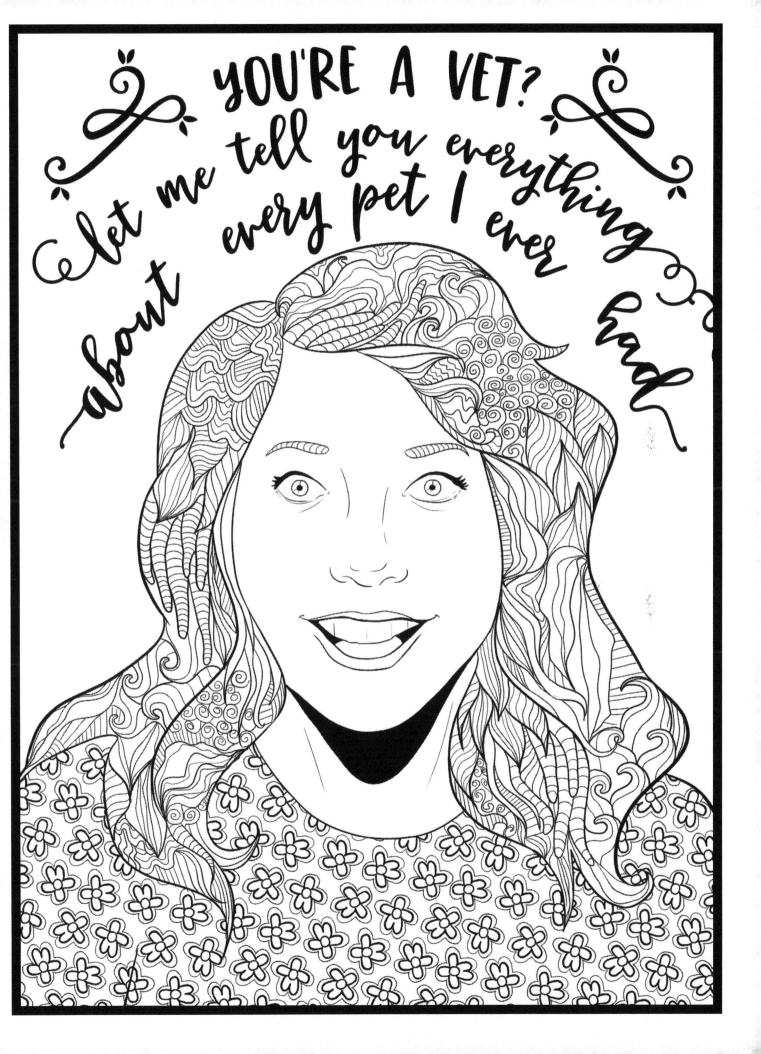

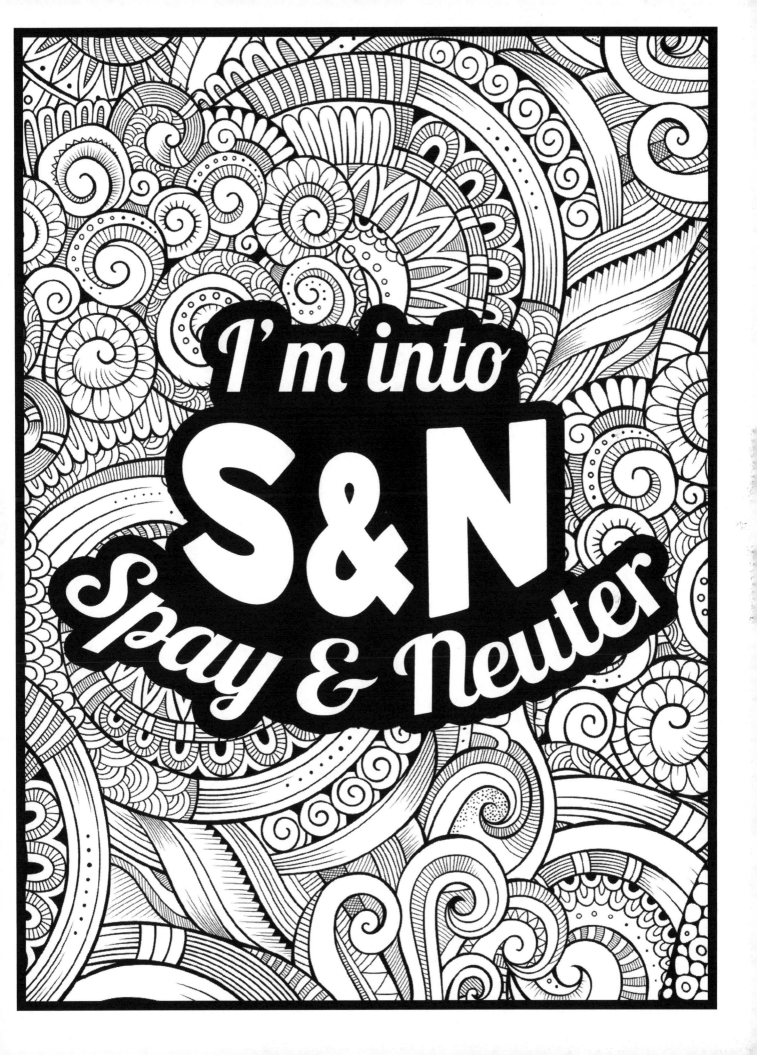

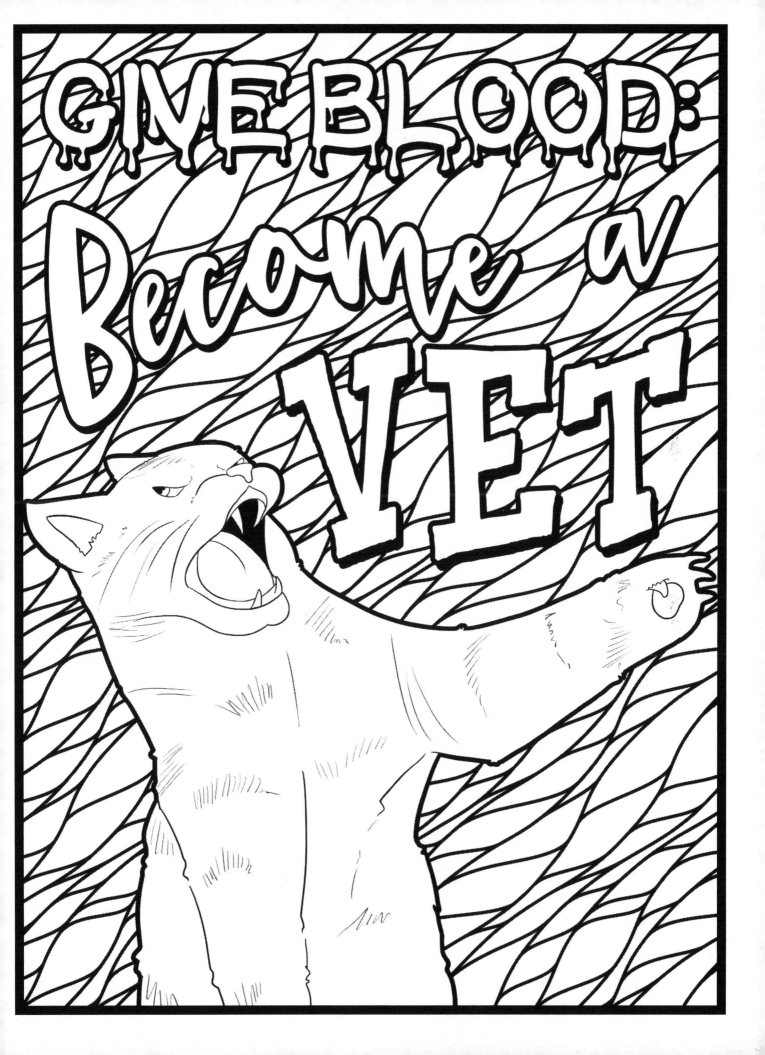

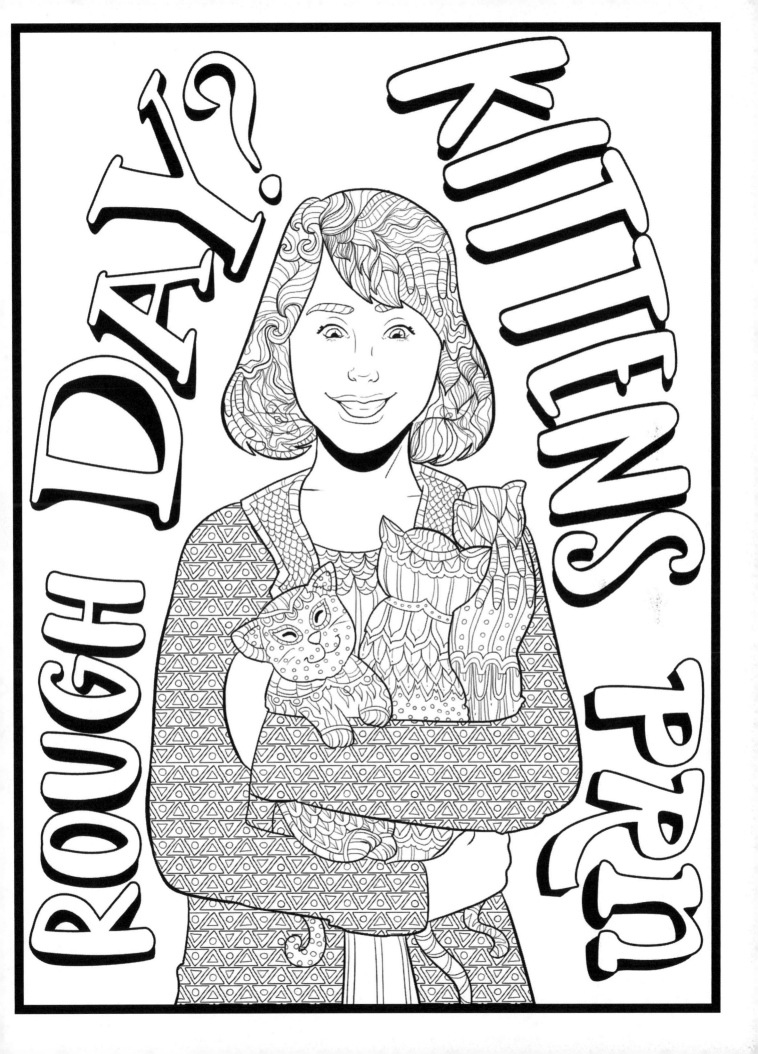

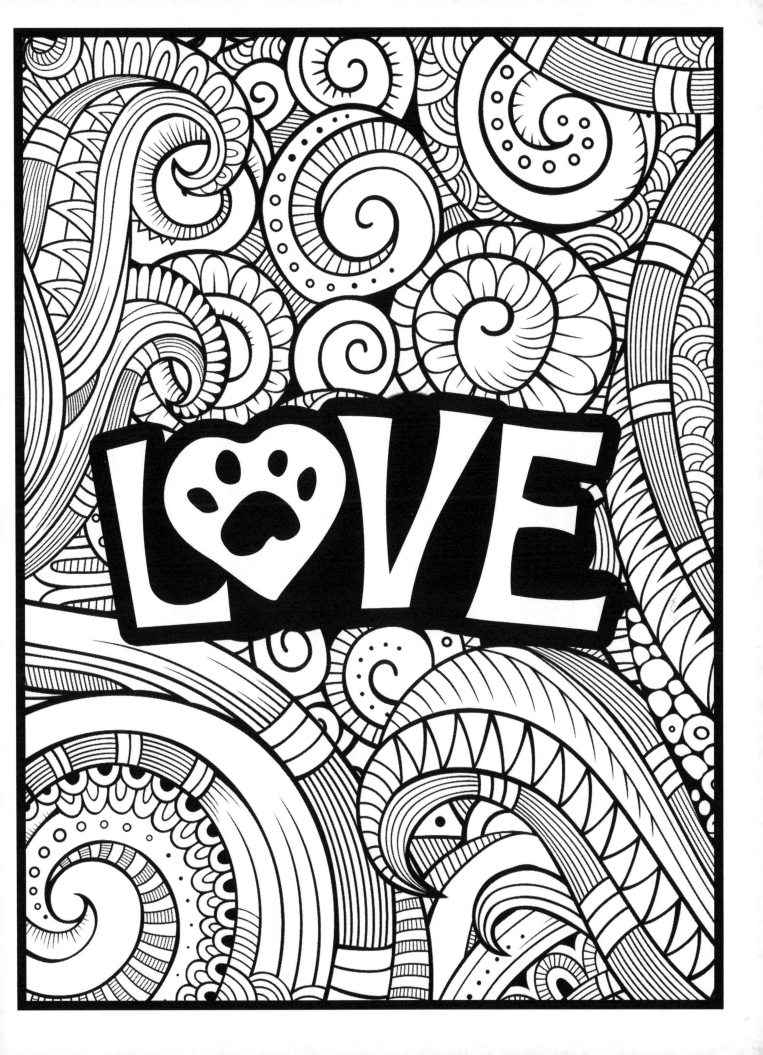

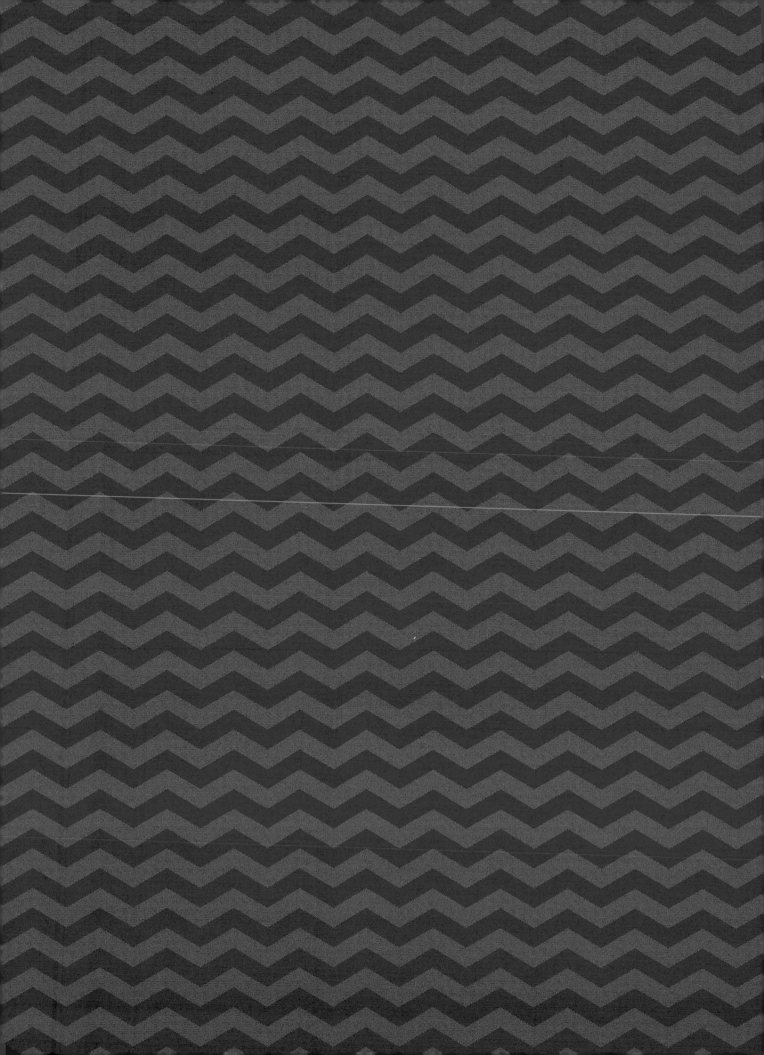

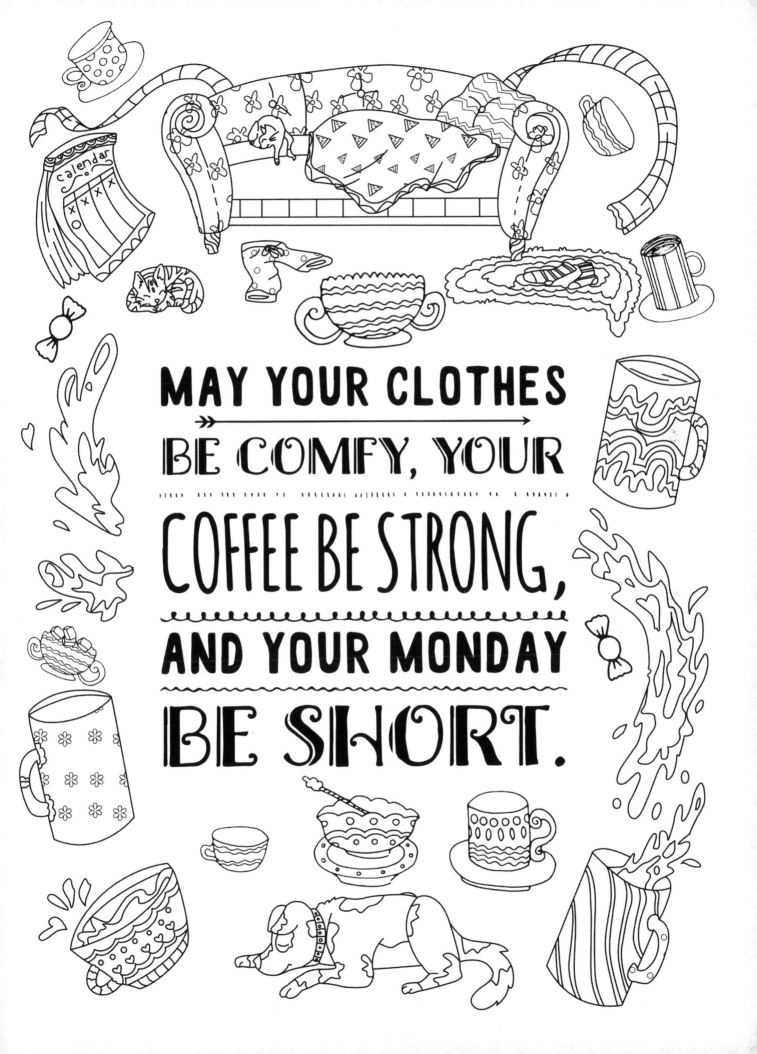

MAY YOUR CLOTHES BE COMFY, YOUR COFFEE BE STRONG, AND YOUR MONDAY BE SHORT.

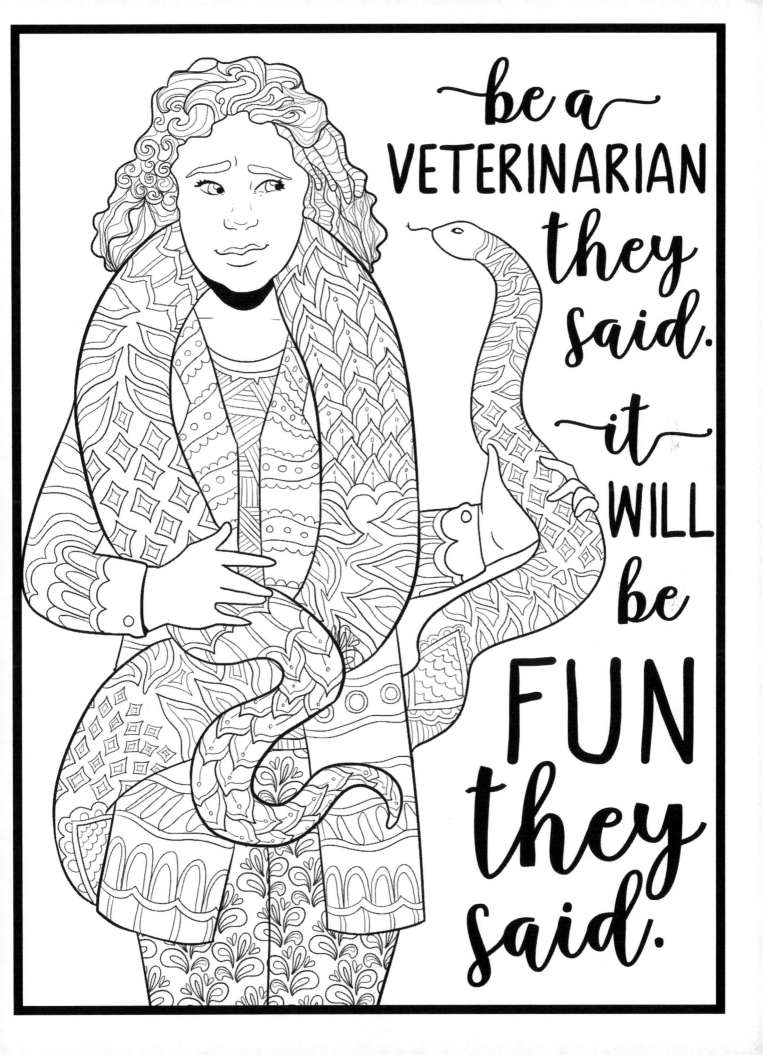

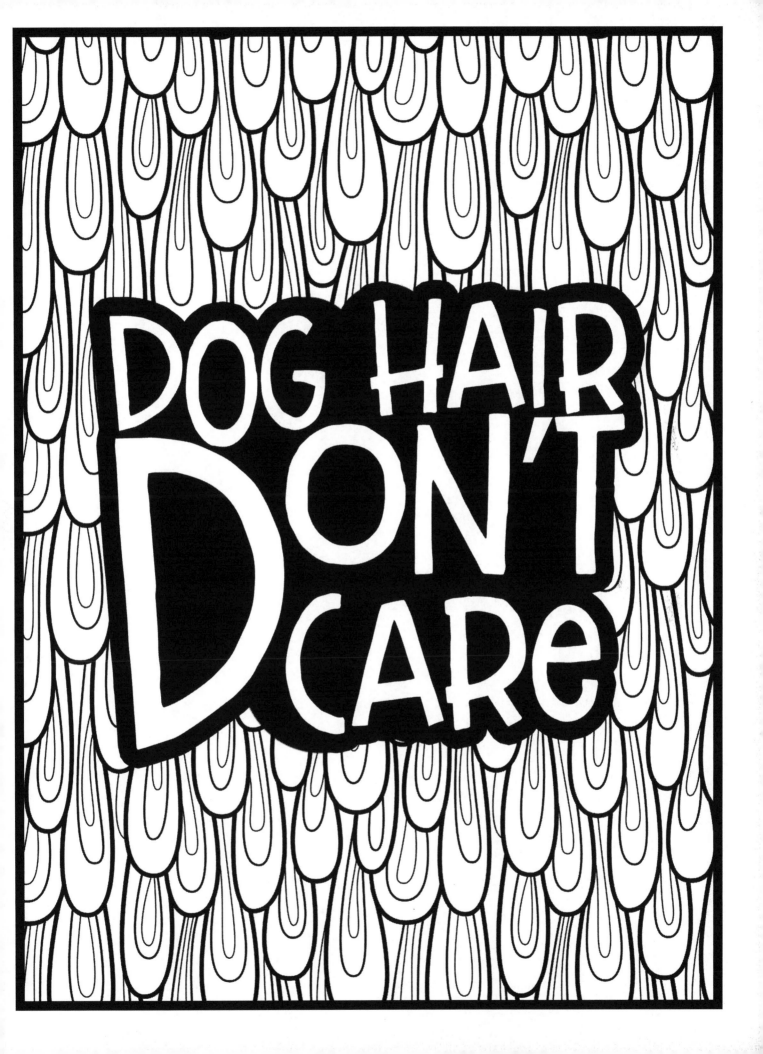

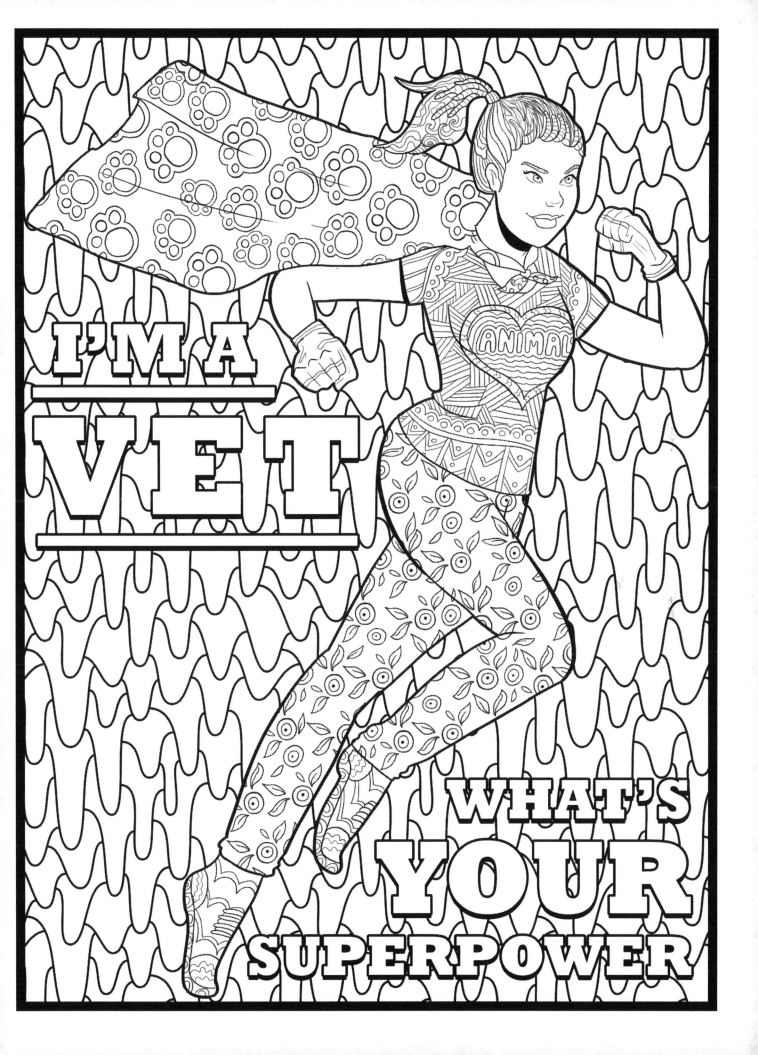

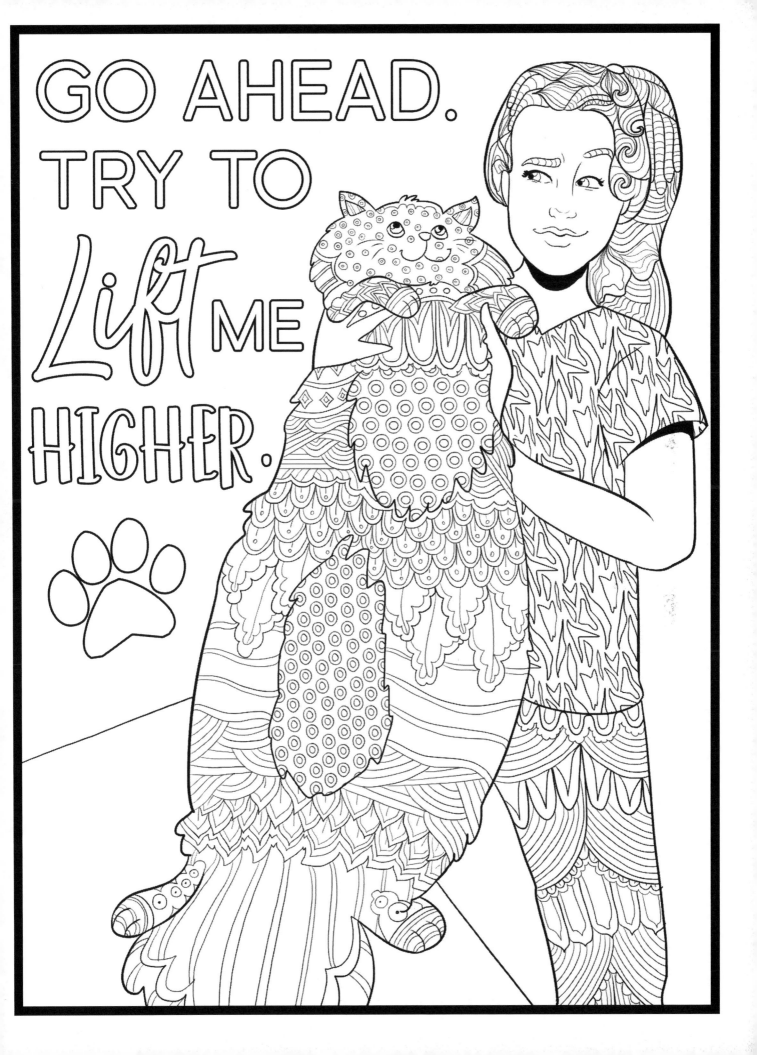

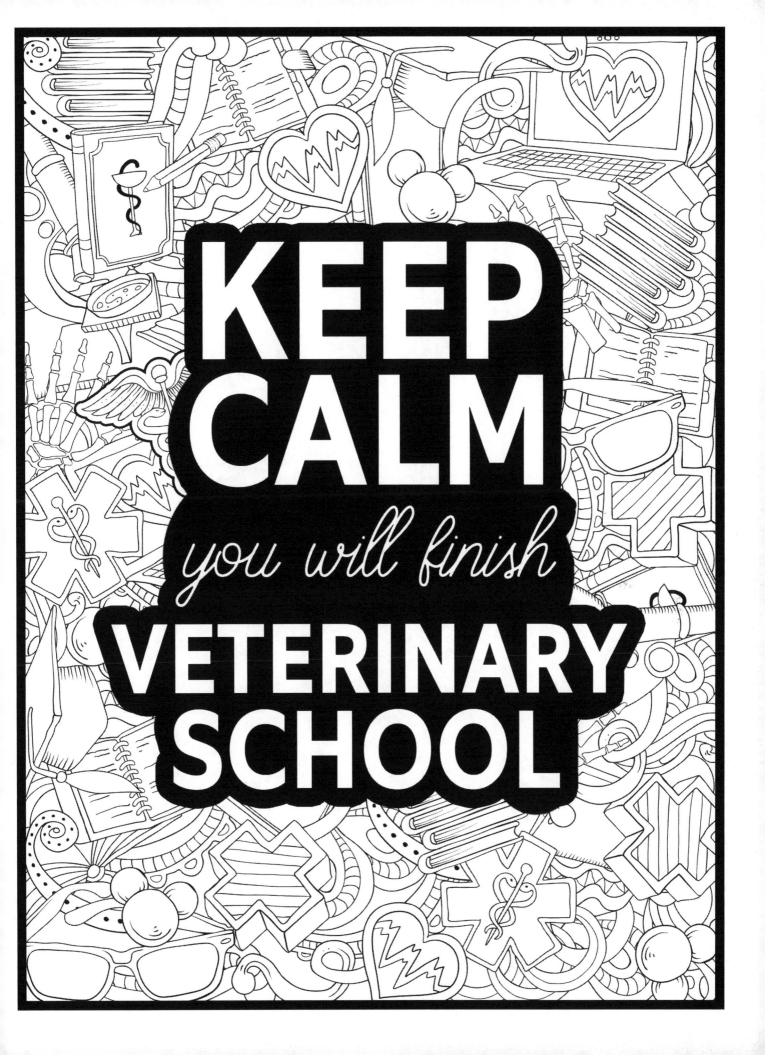

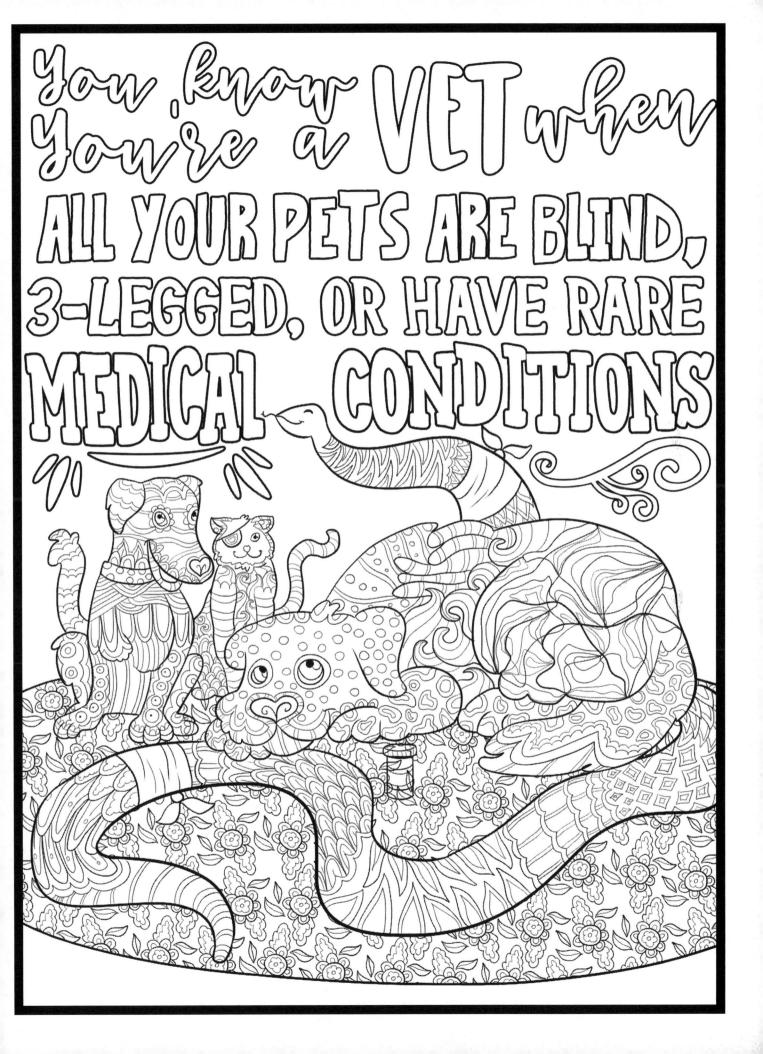

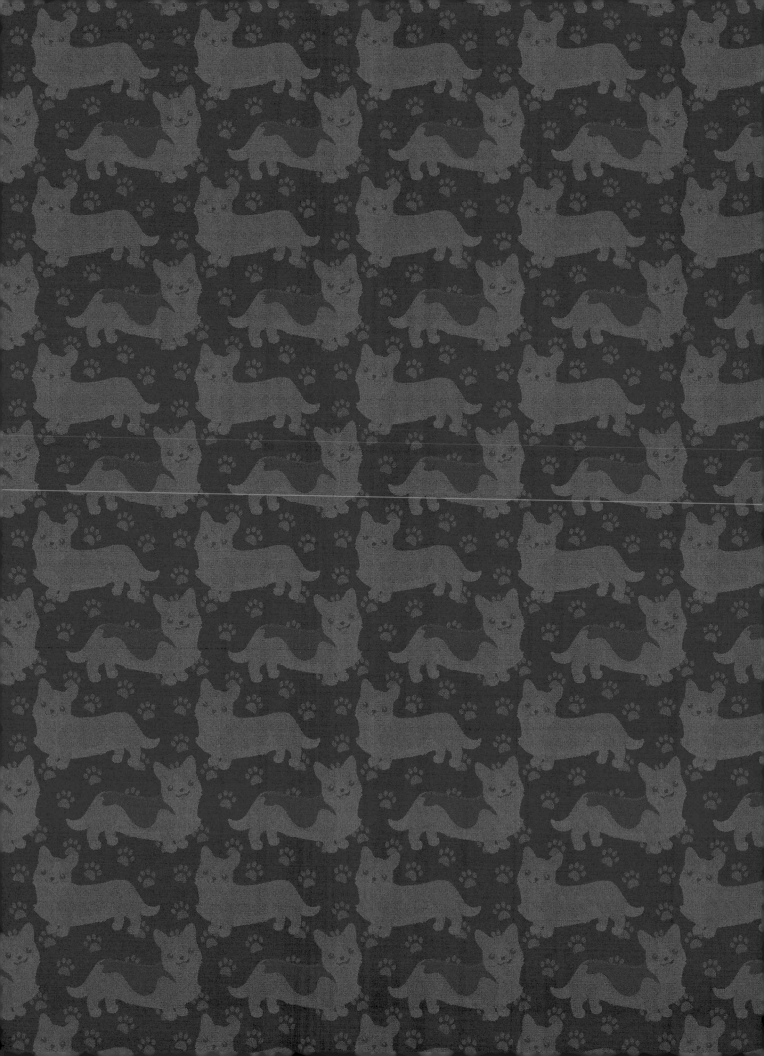

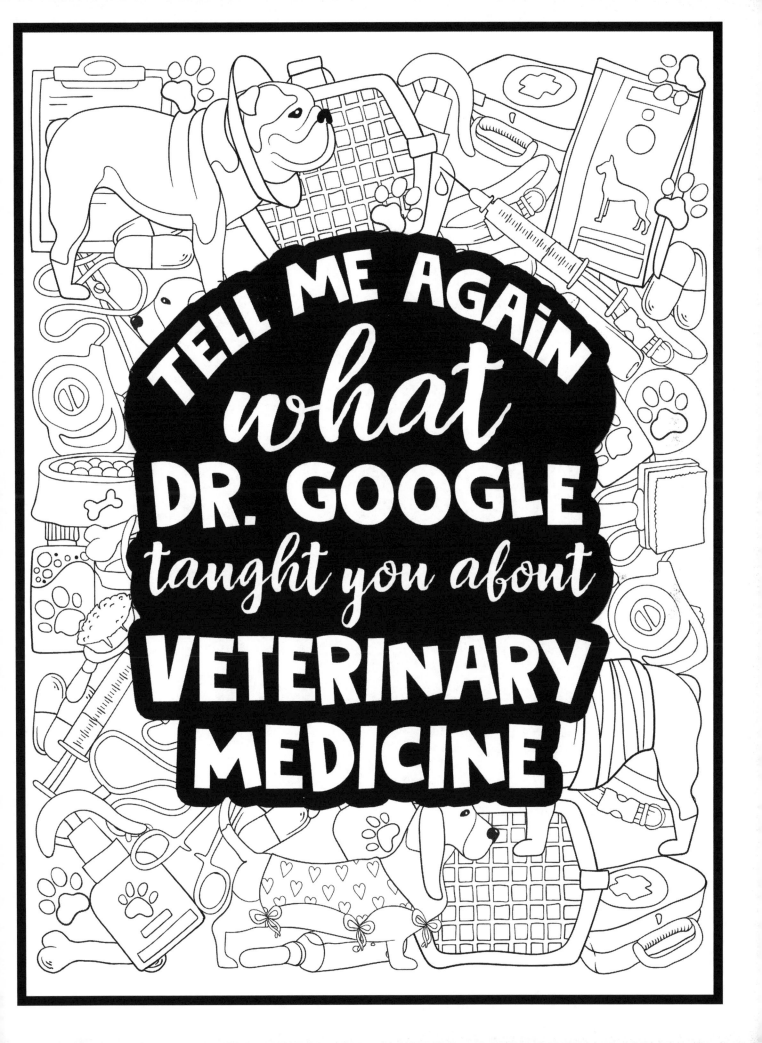

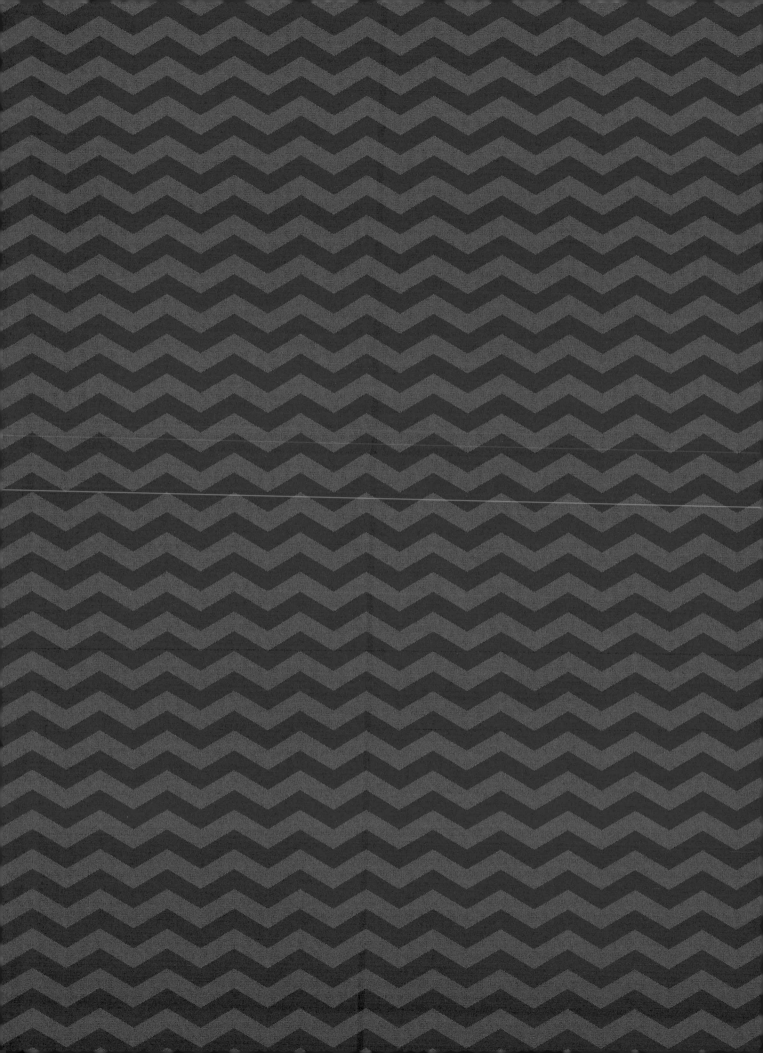

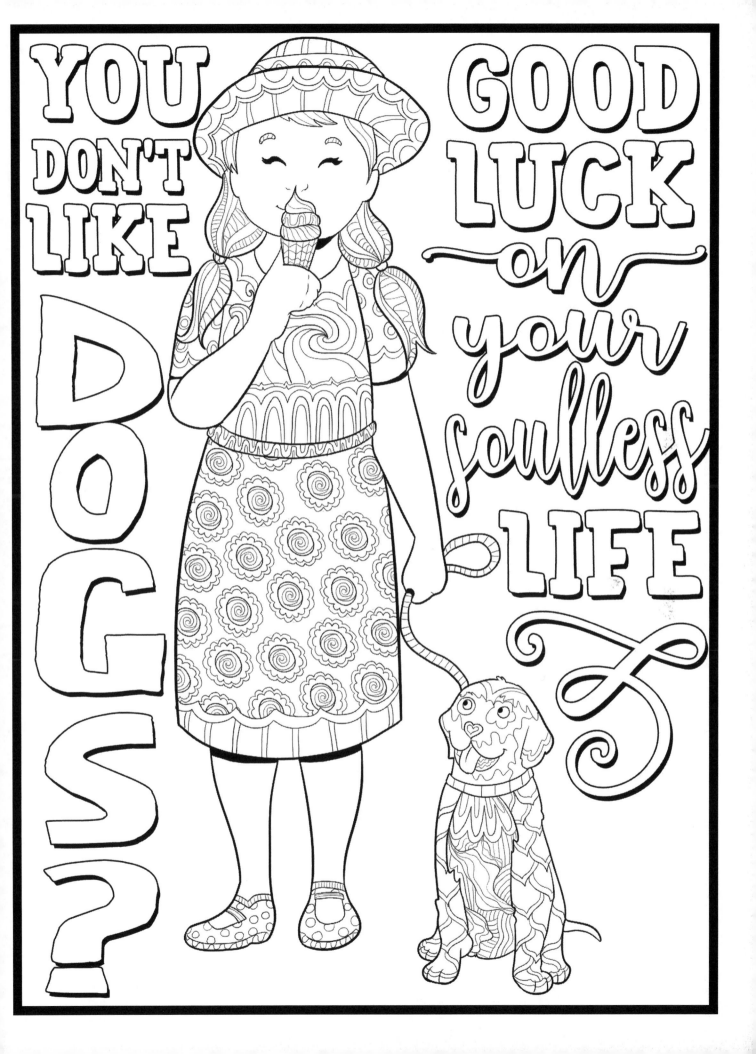

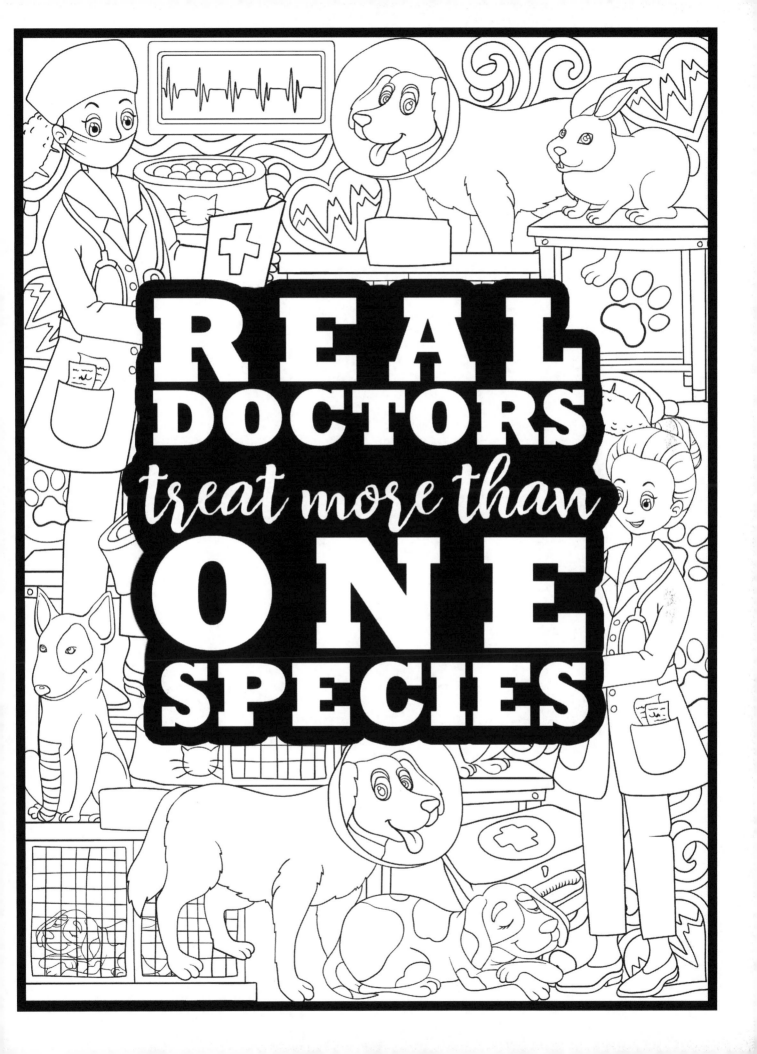

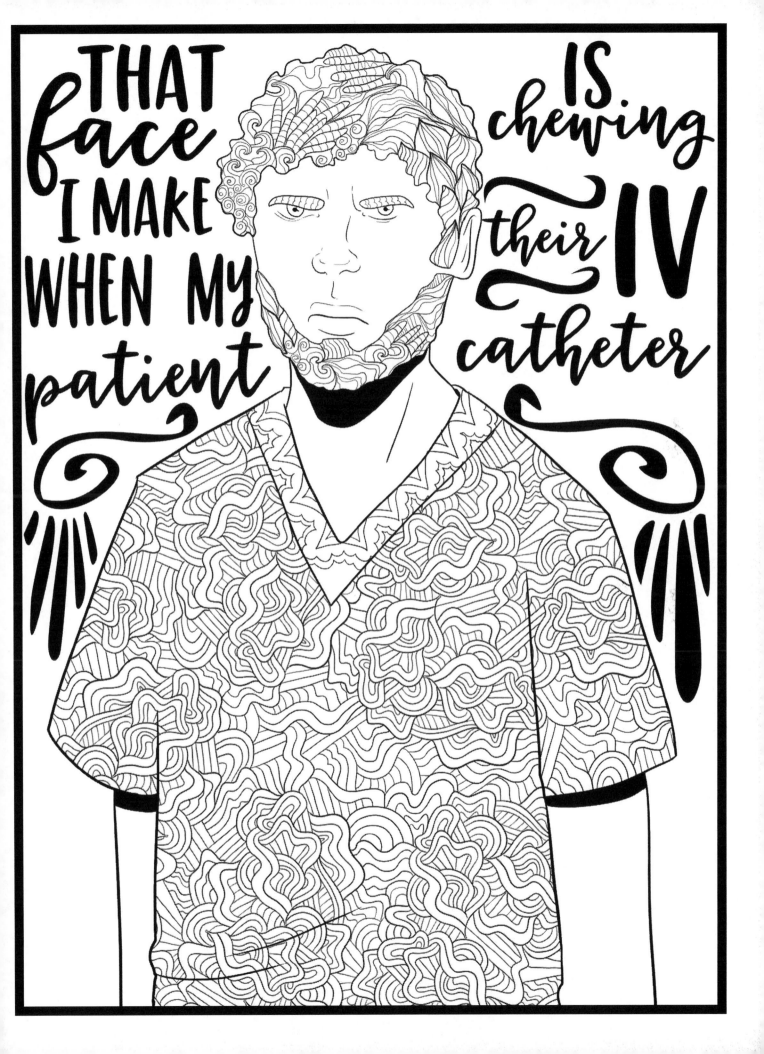

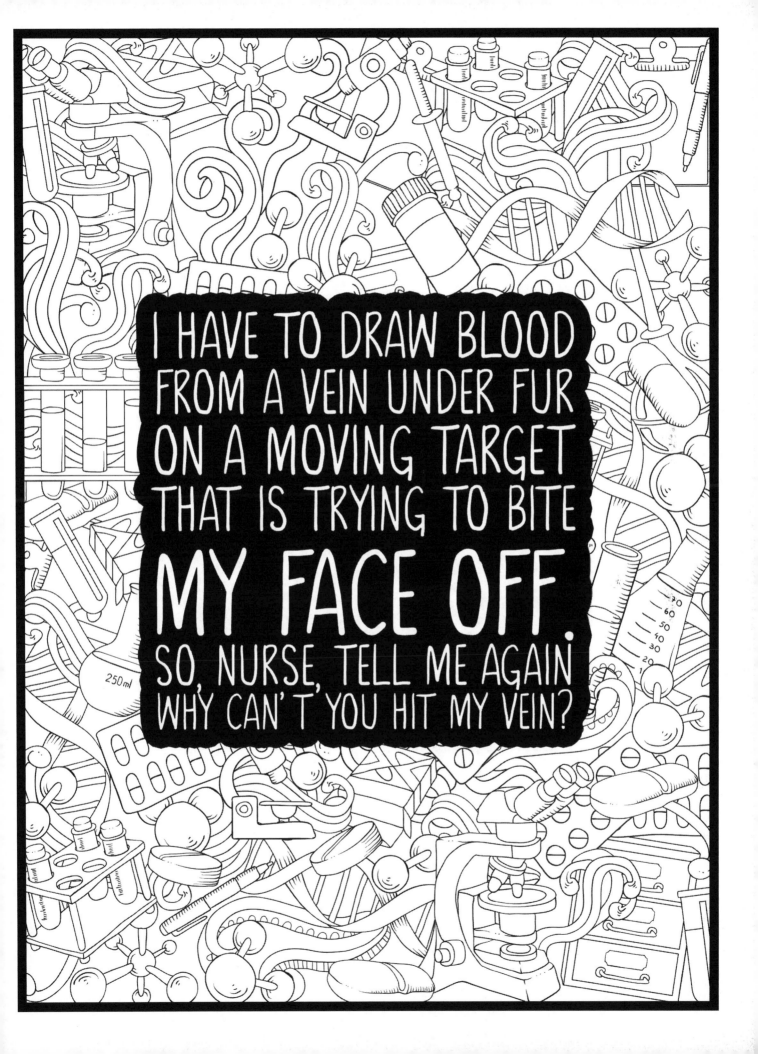

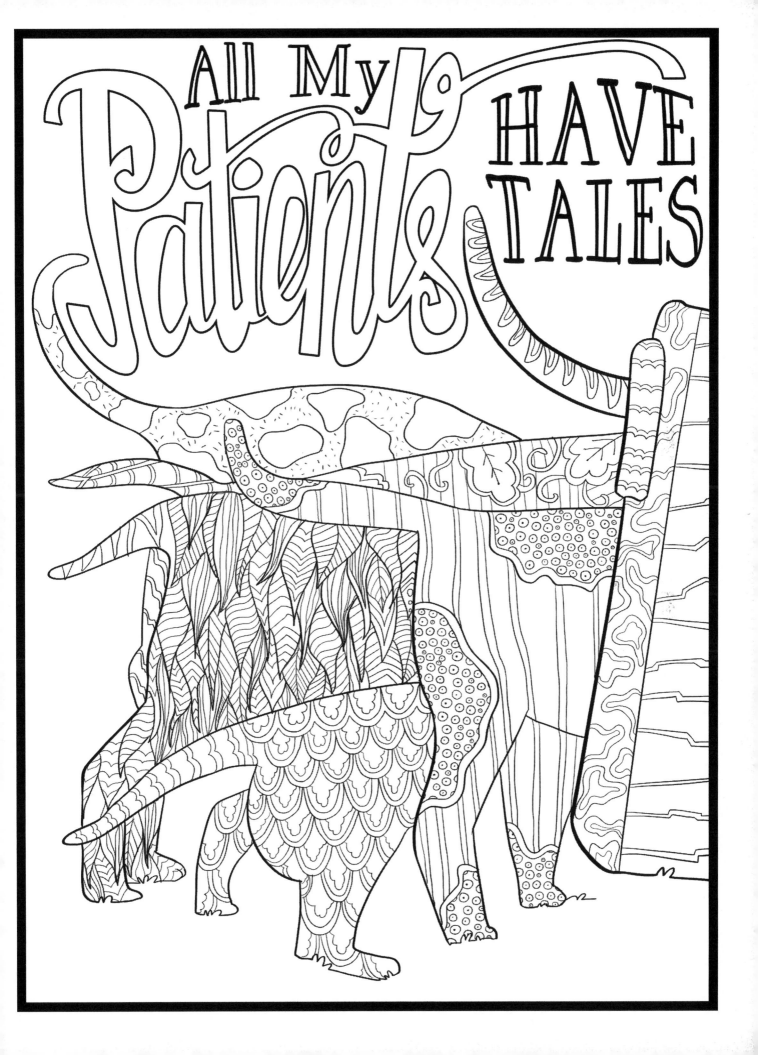

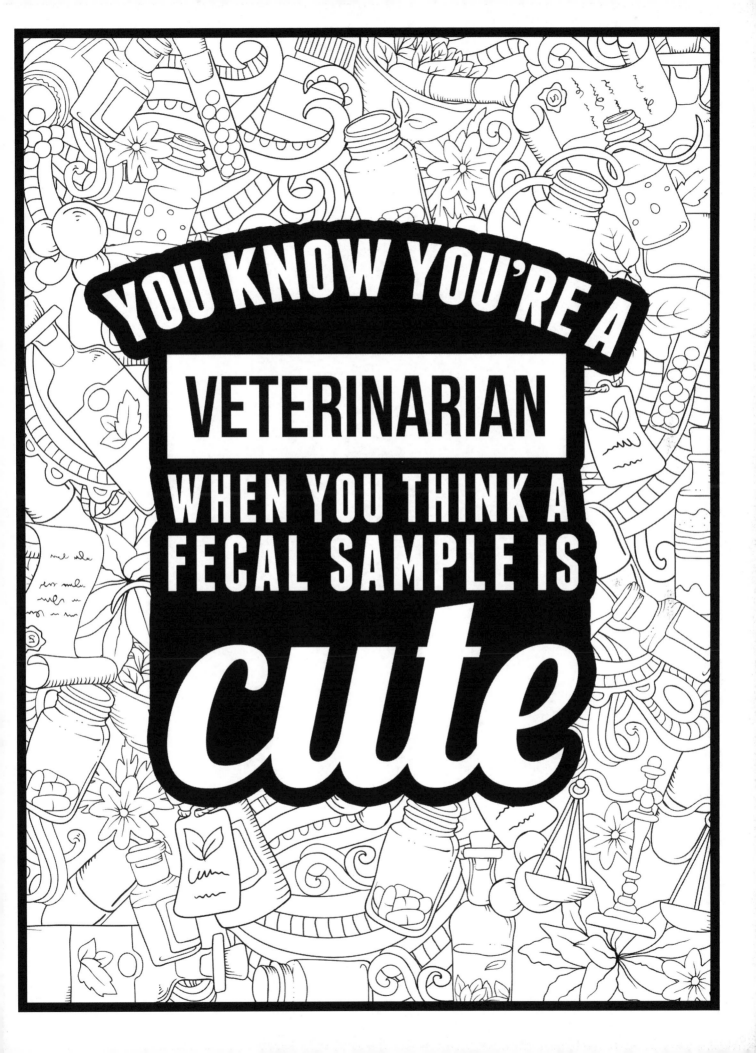

I JUST WANT TO DRINK COFFEE SAVE ANIMALS AND TAKE NAPS

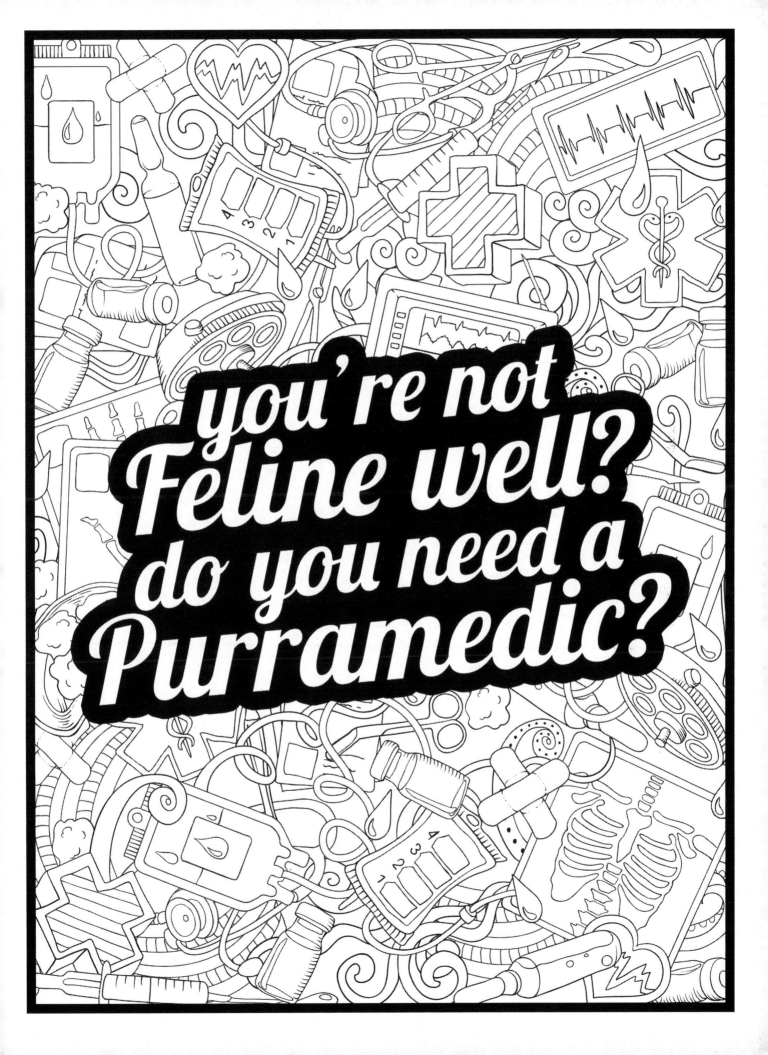

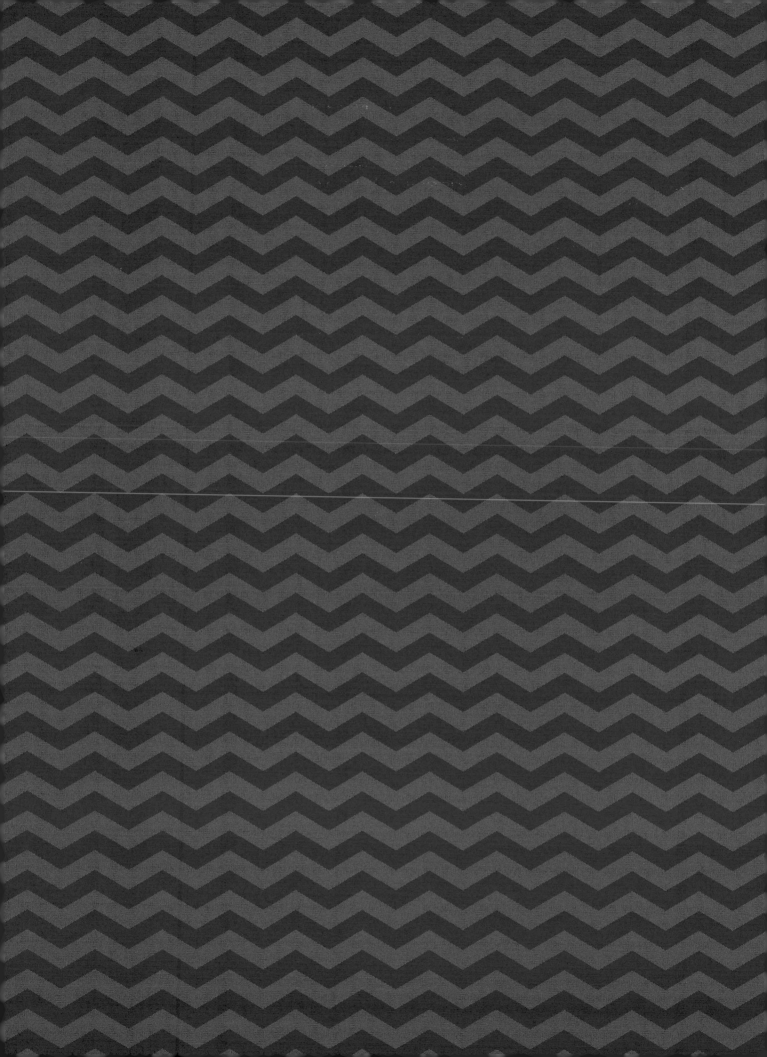

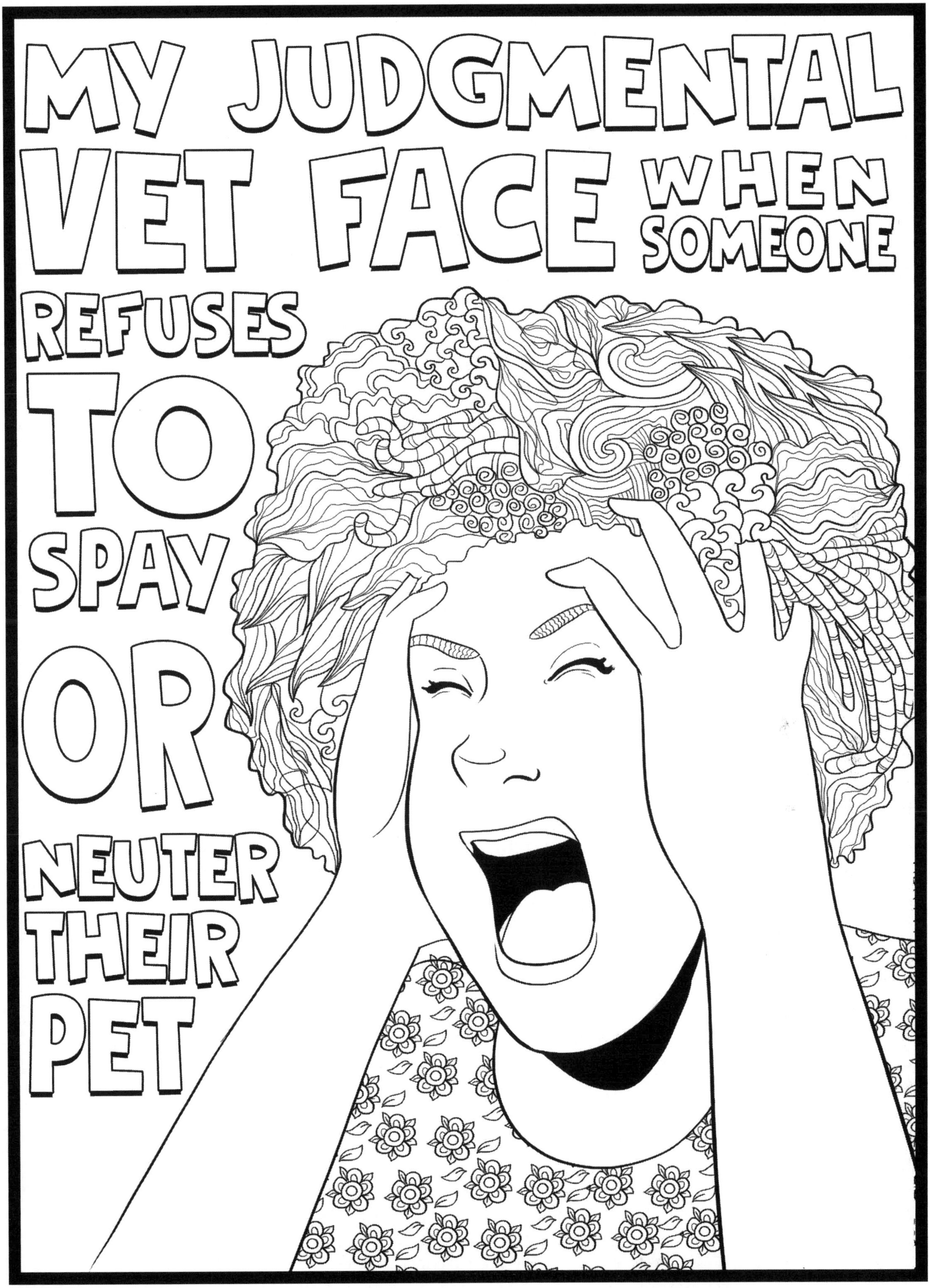
MY JUDGMENTAL VET FACE WHEN SOMEONE REFUSES TO SPAY OR NEUTER THEIR PET

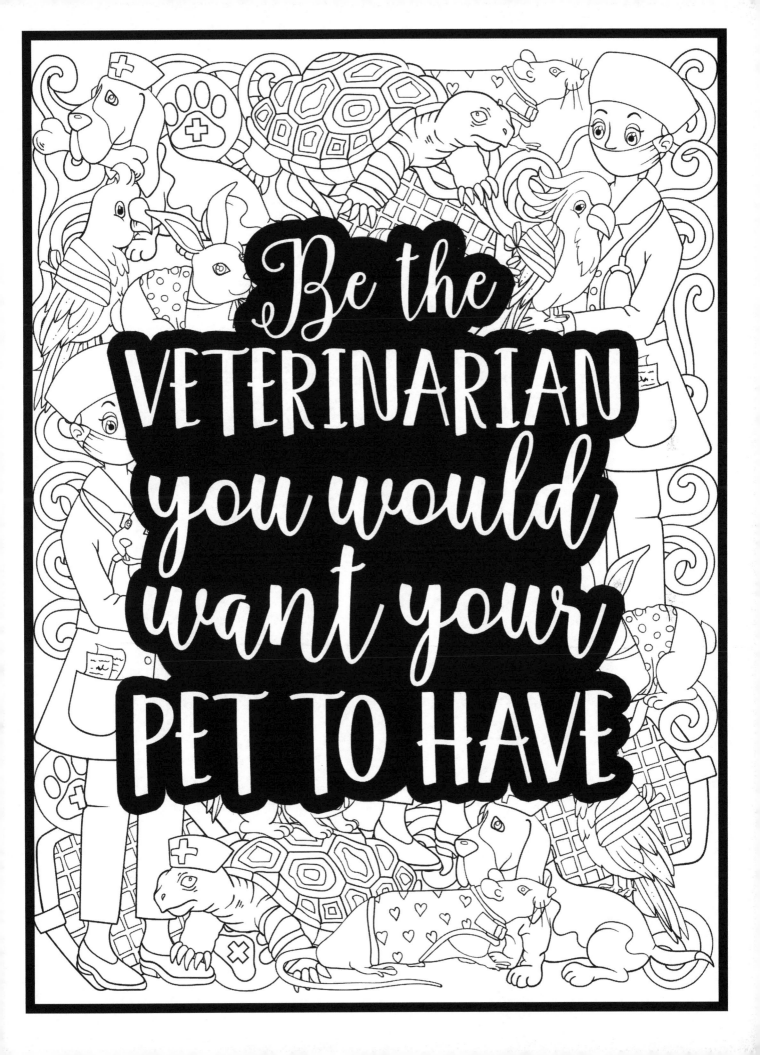

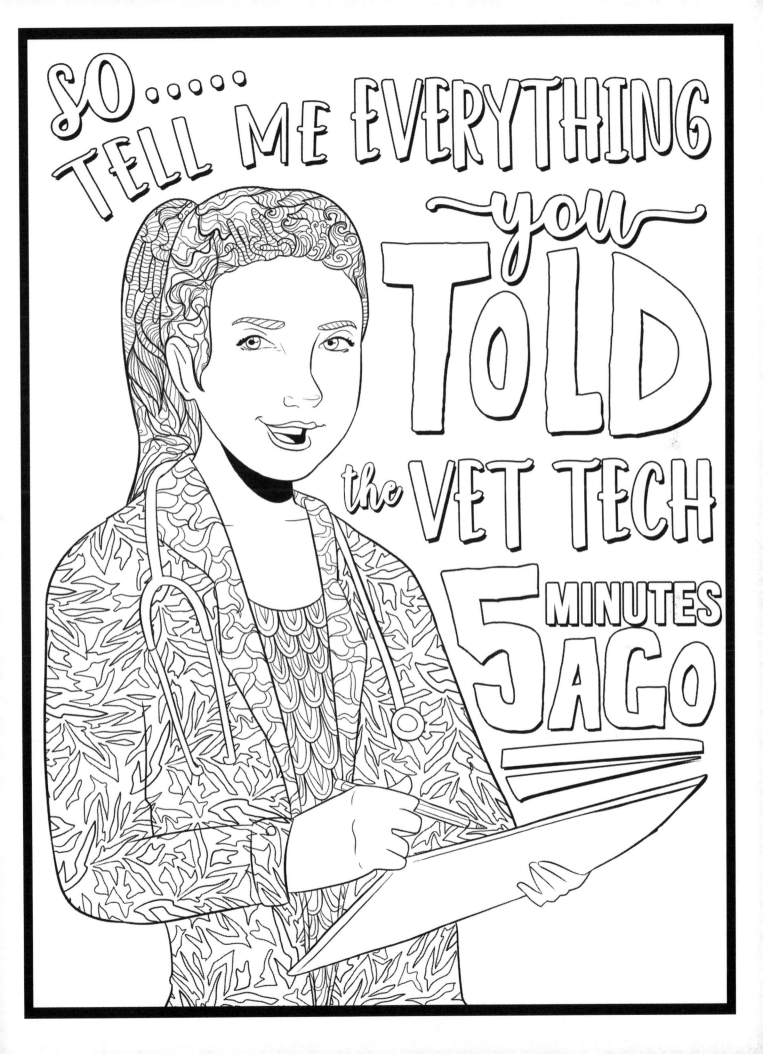

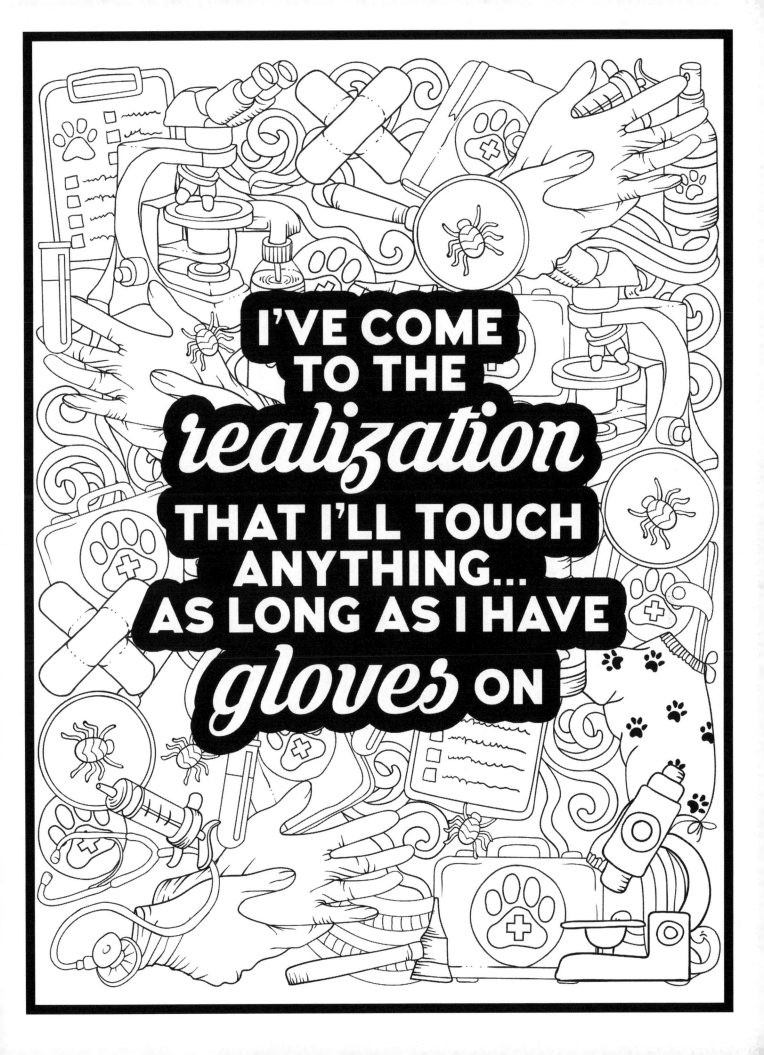

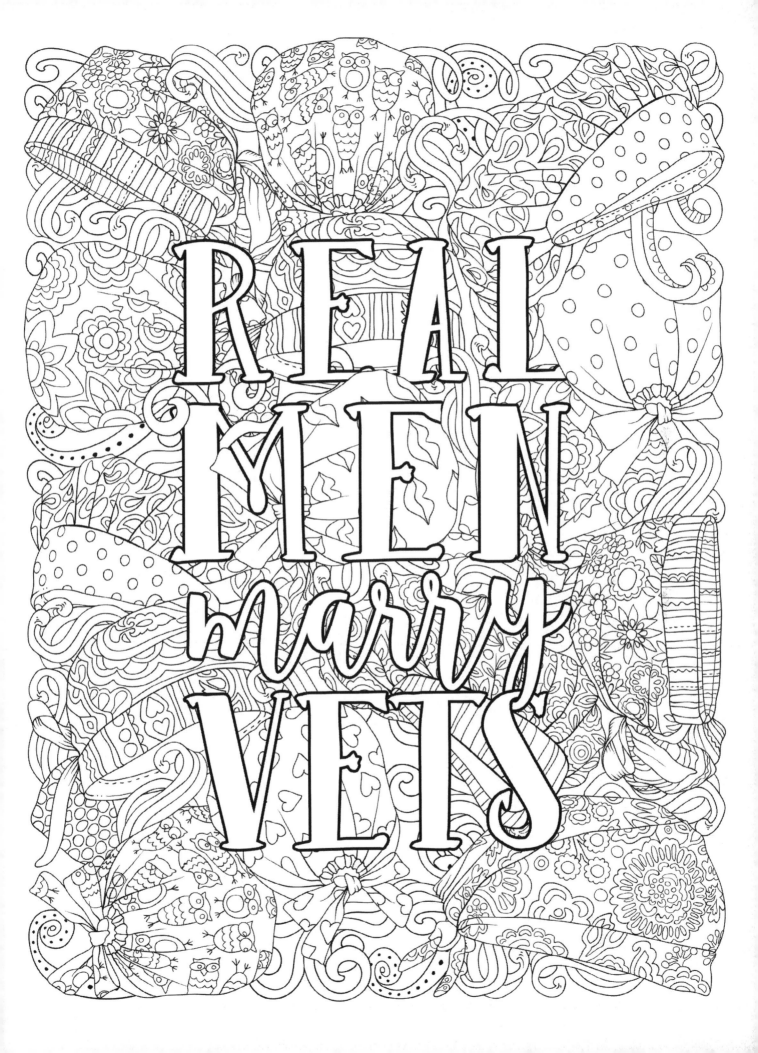

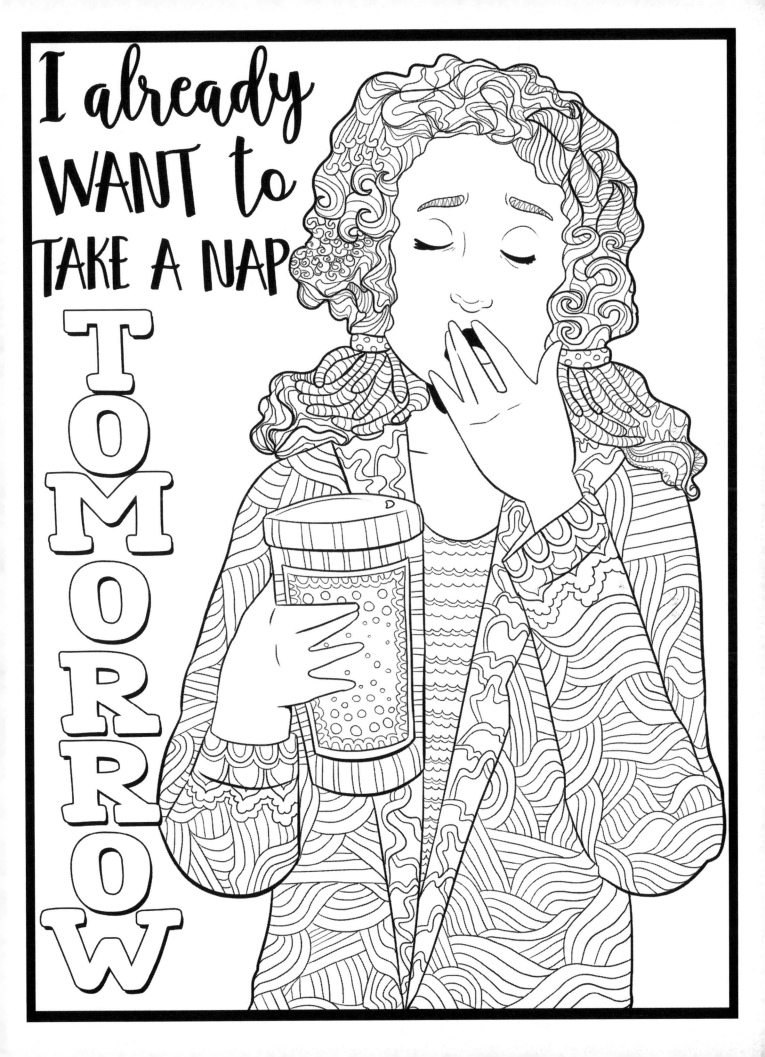

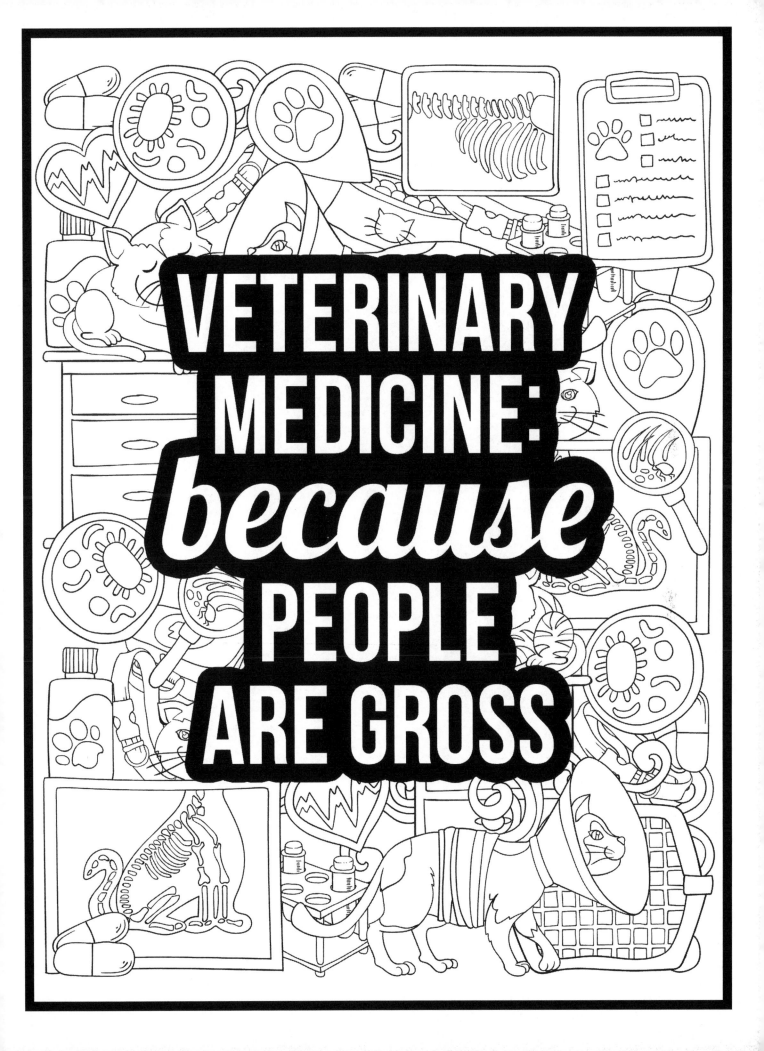

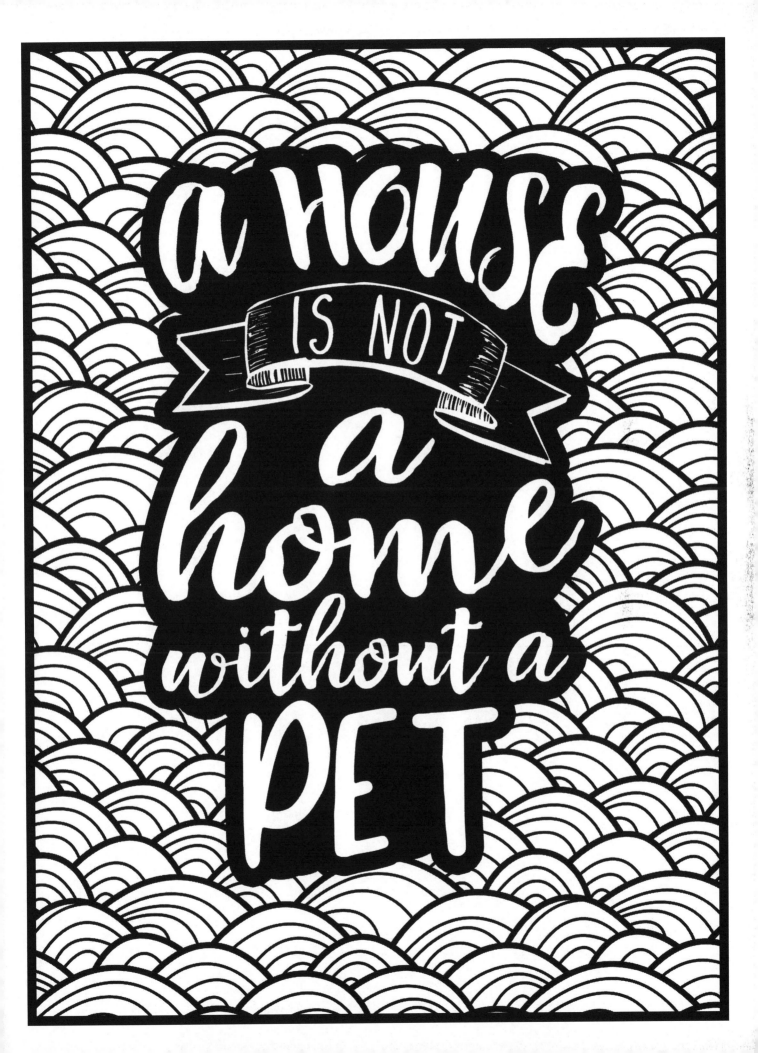

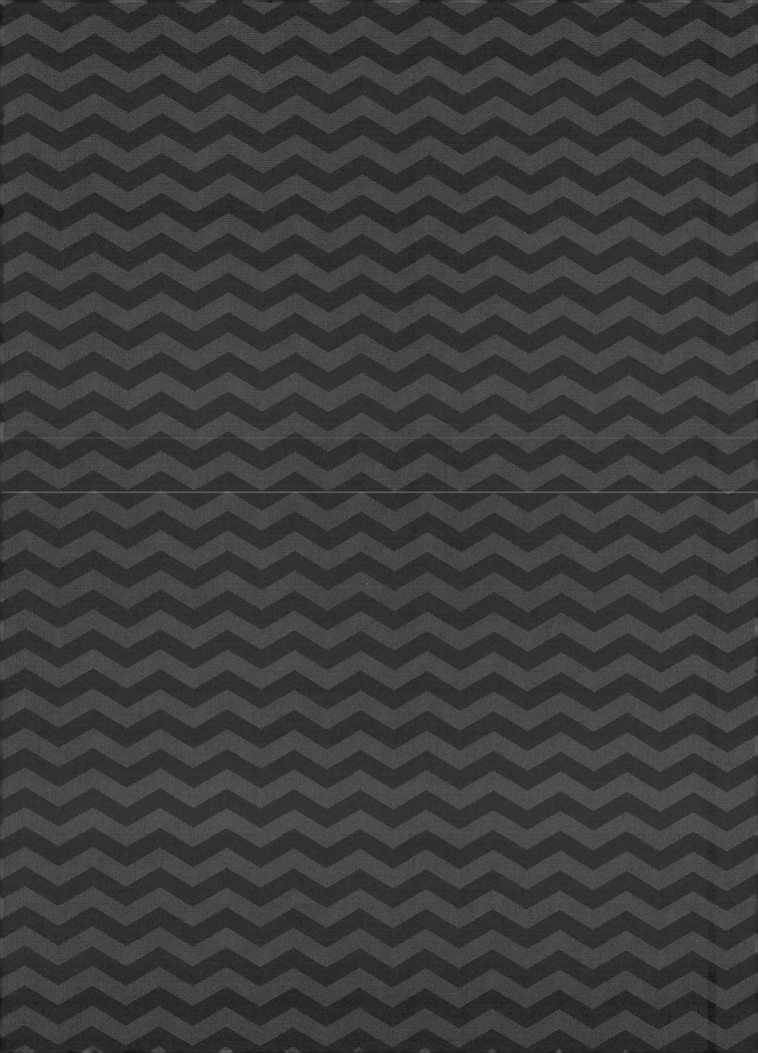

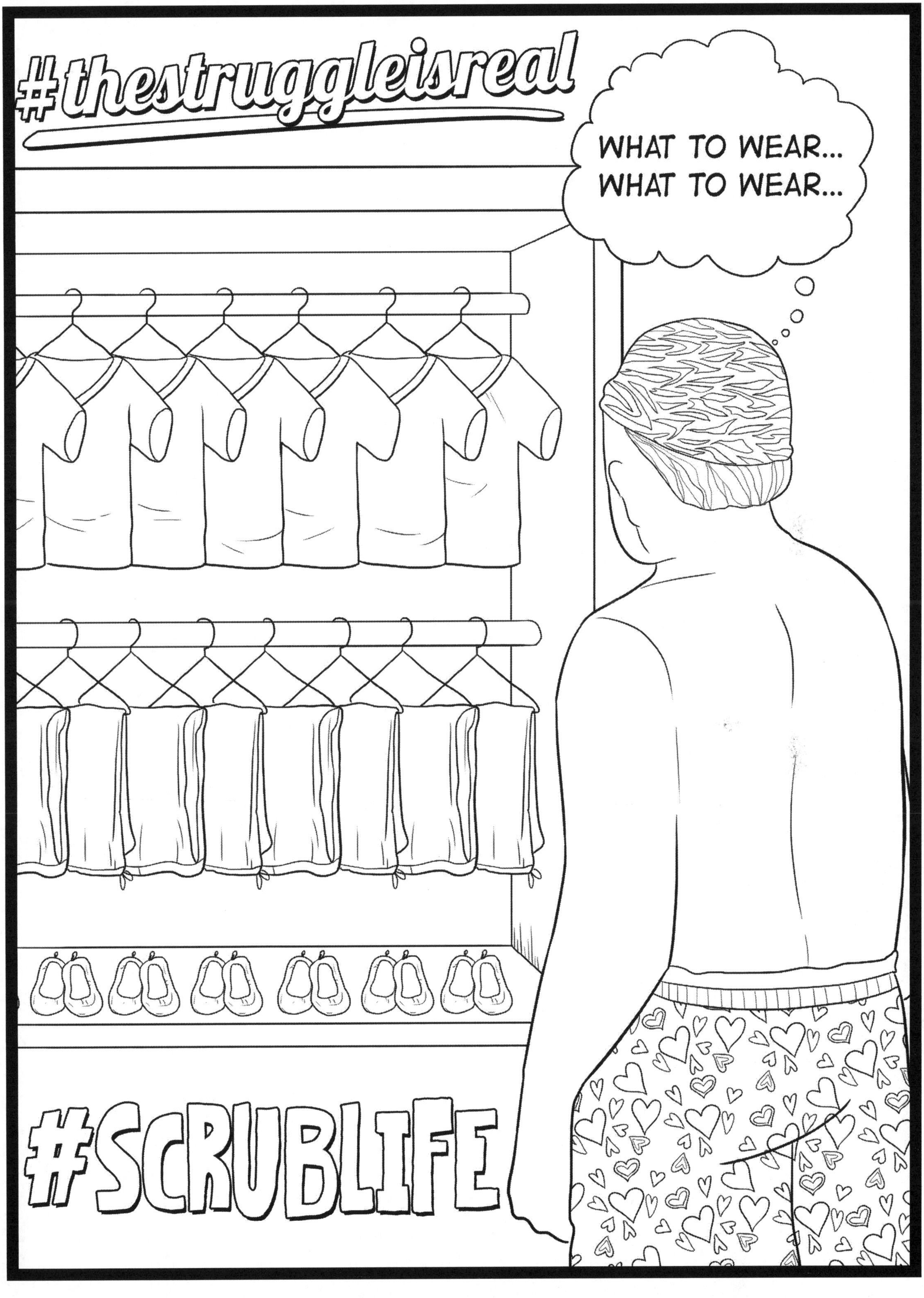
#thestruggleisreal
WHAT TO WEAR... WHAT TO WEAR...
#SCRUBLIFE

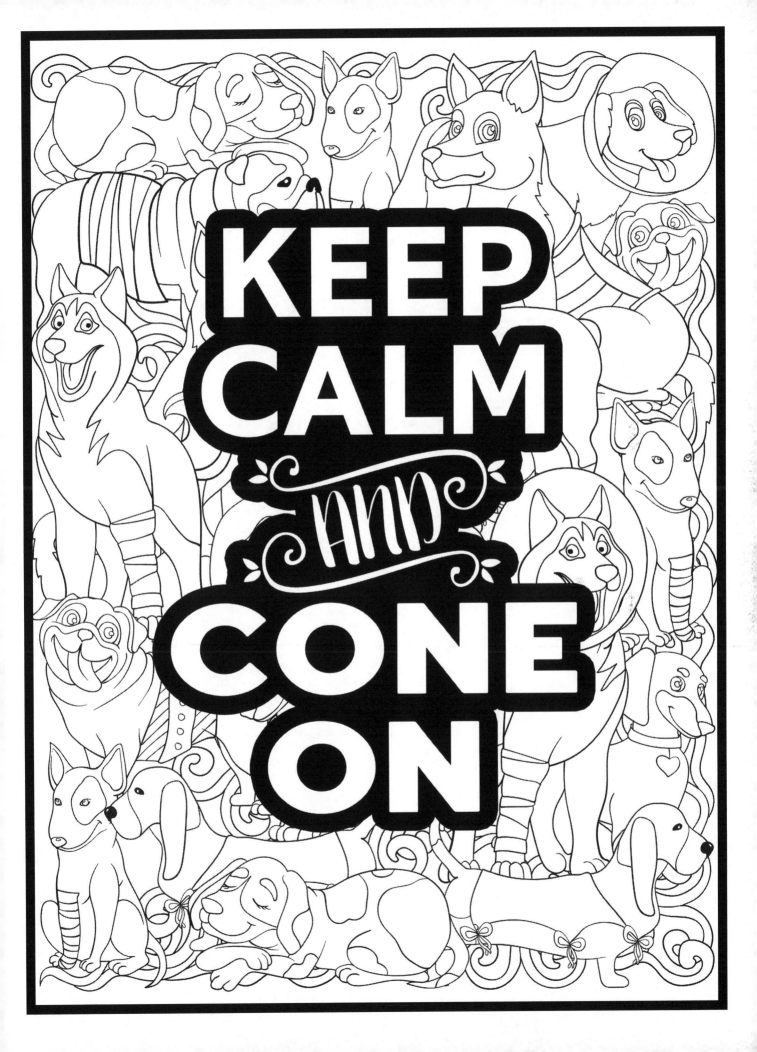

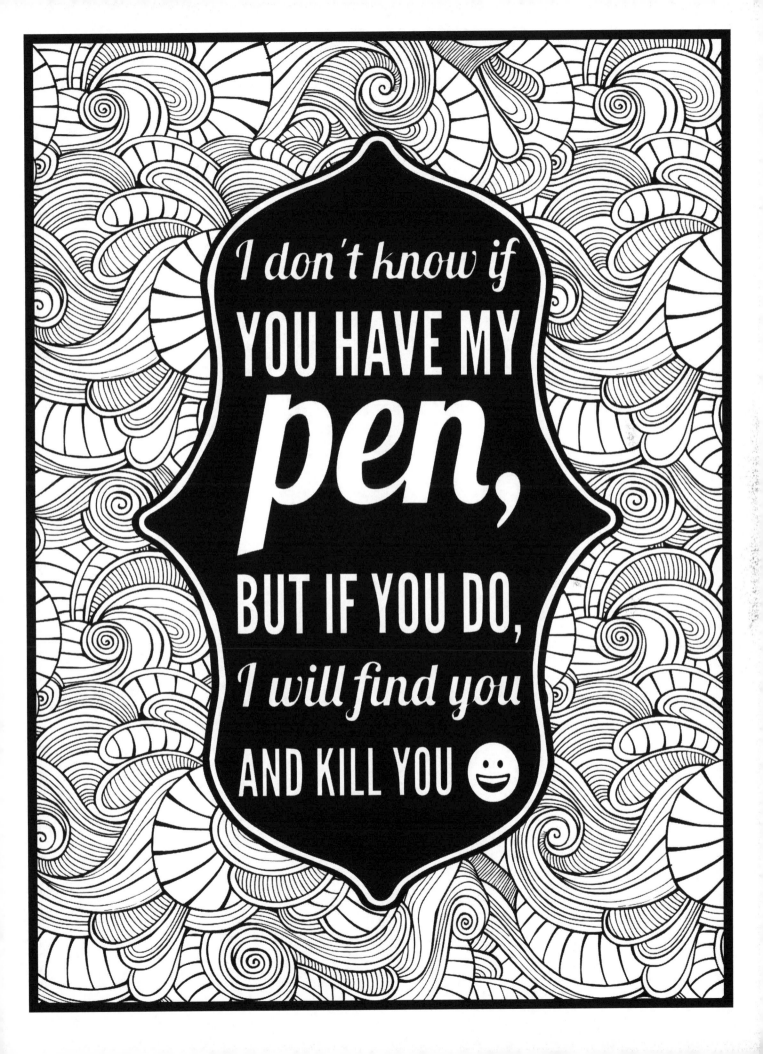

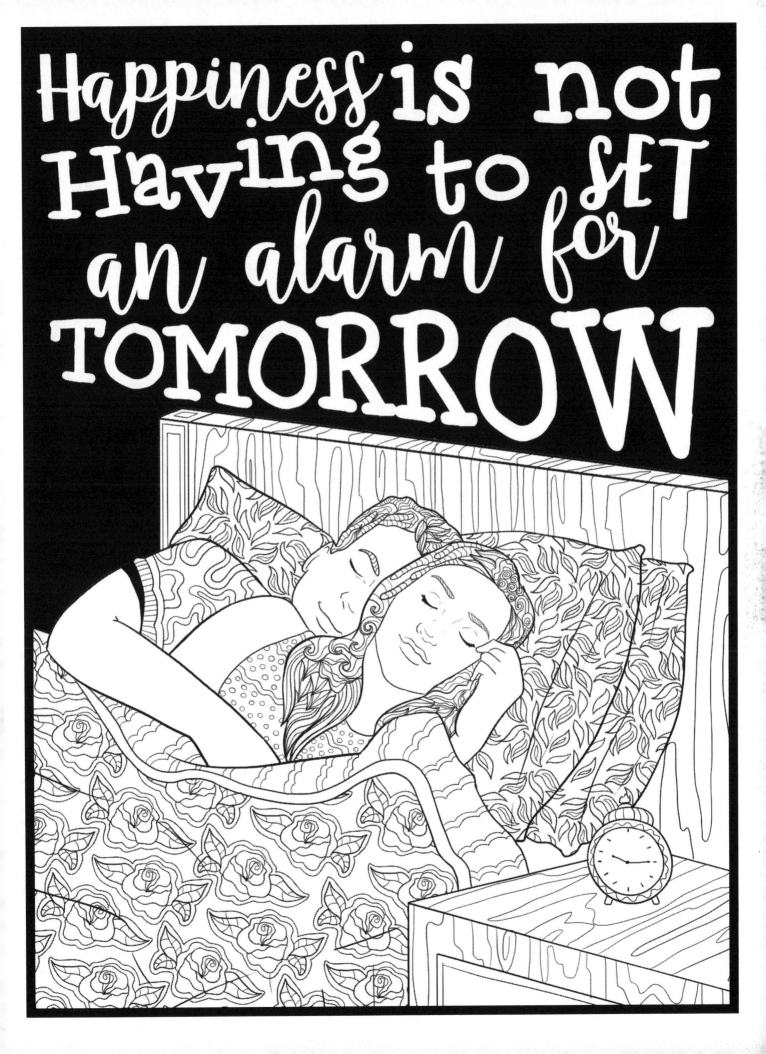

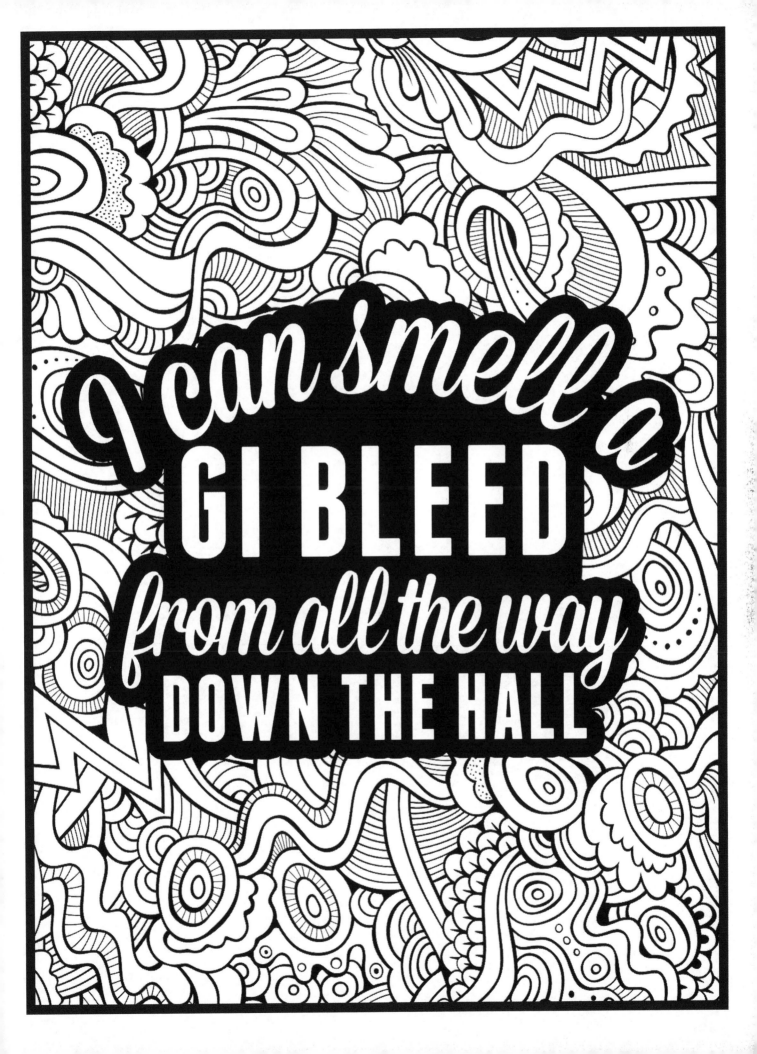

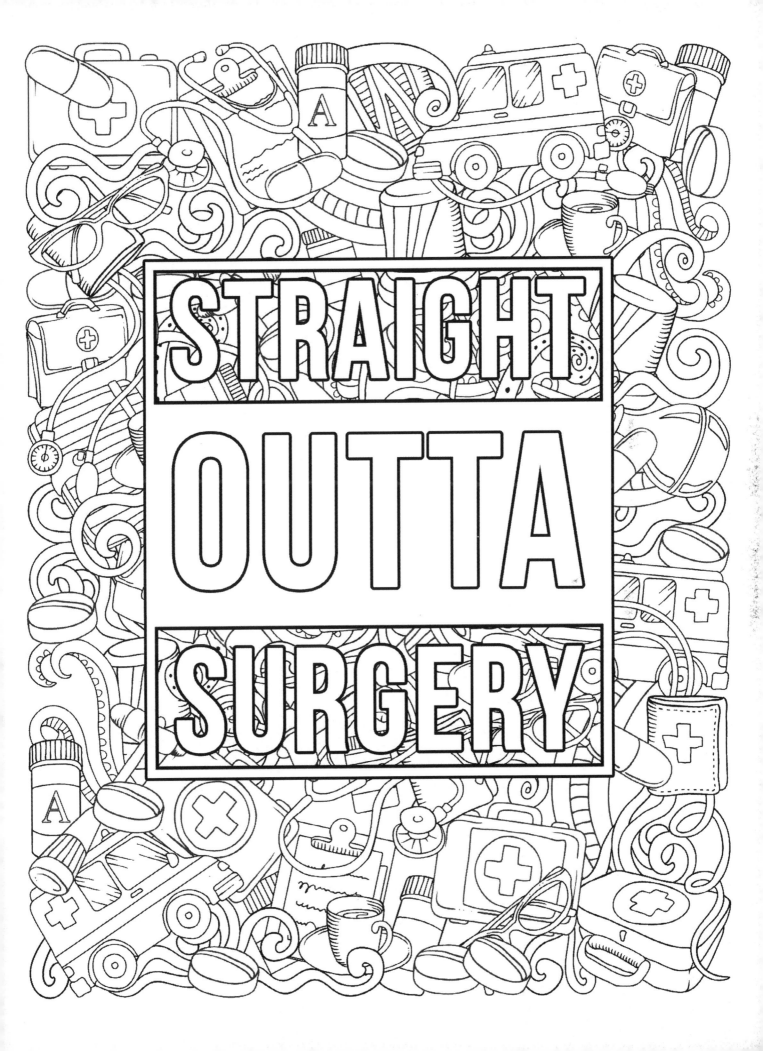

VET SCHOOL IS LIKE RIDING A BIKE. EXCEPT THE BIKE IS ON FIRE AND YOU'RE ON FIRE AND EVERYTHING IS ON FIRE BECAUSE YOU'RE IN HELL

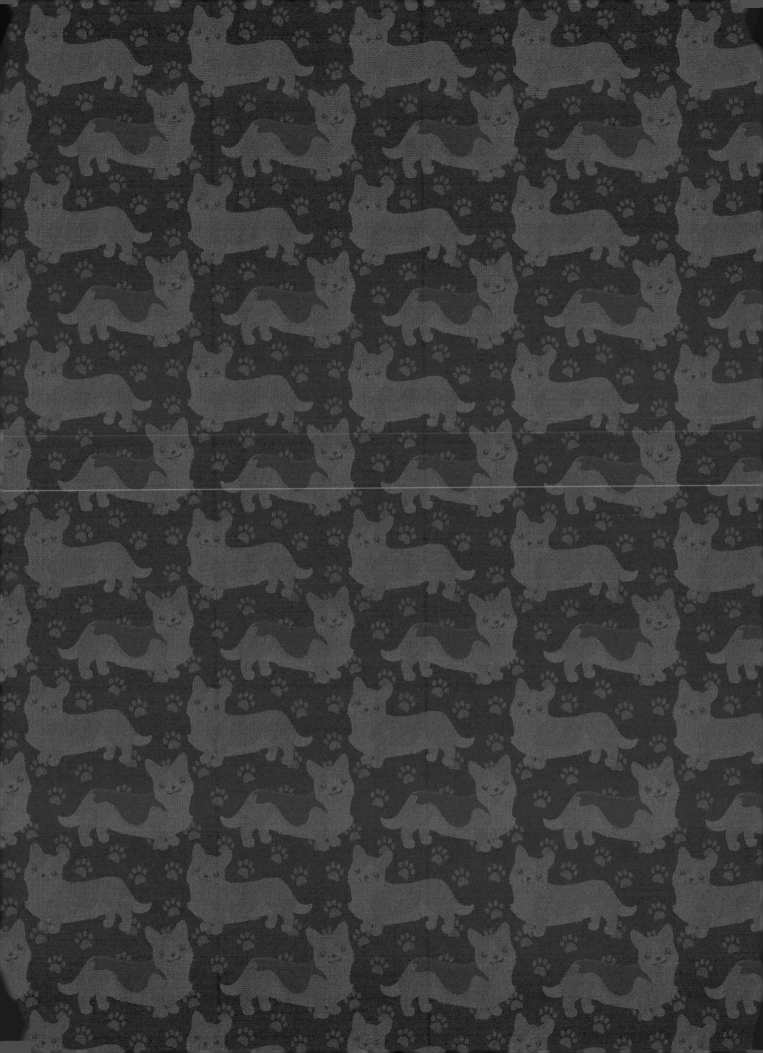

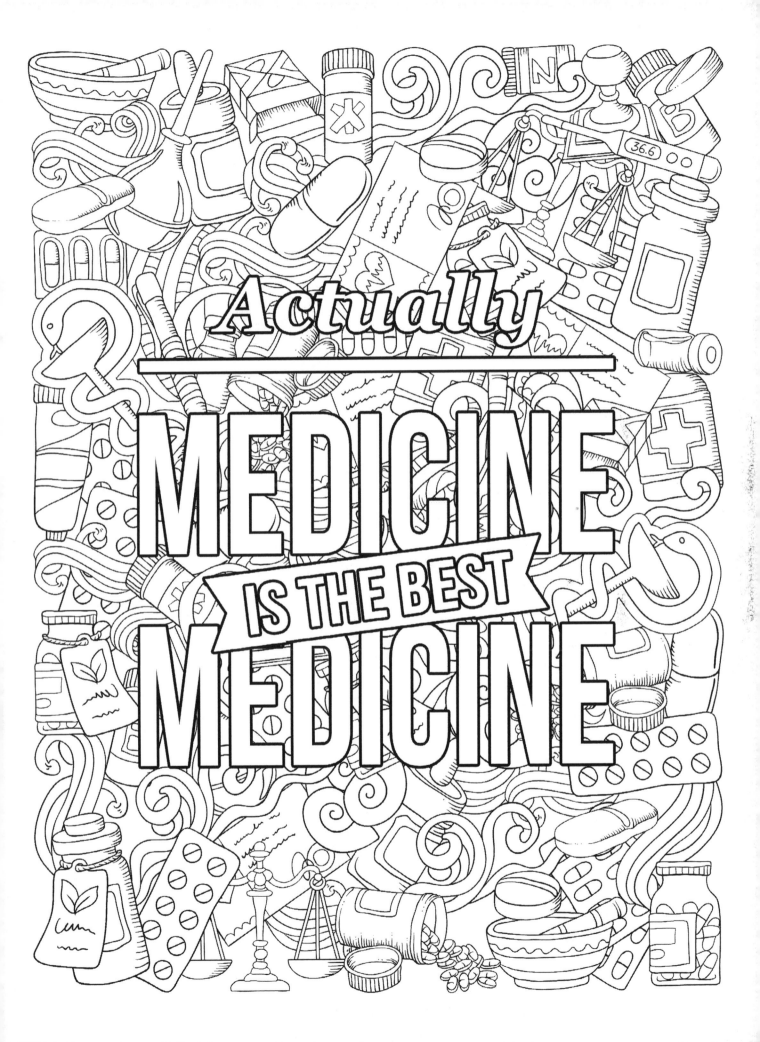

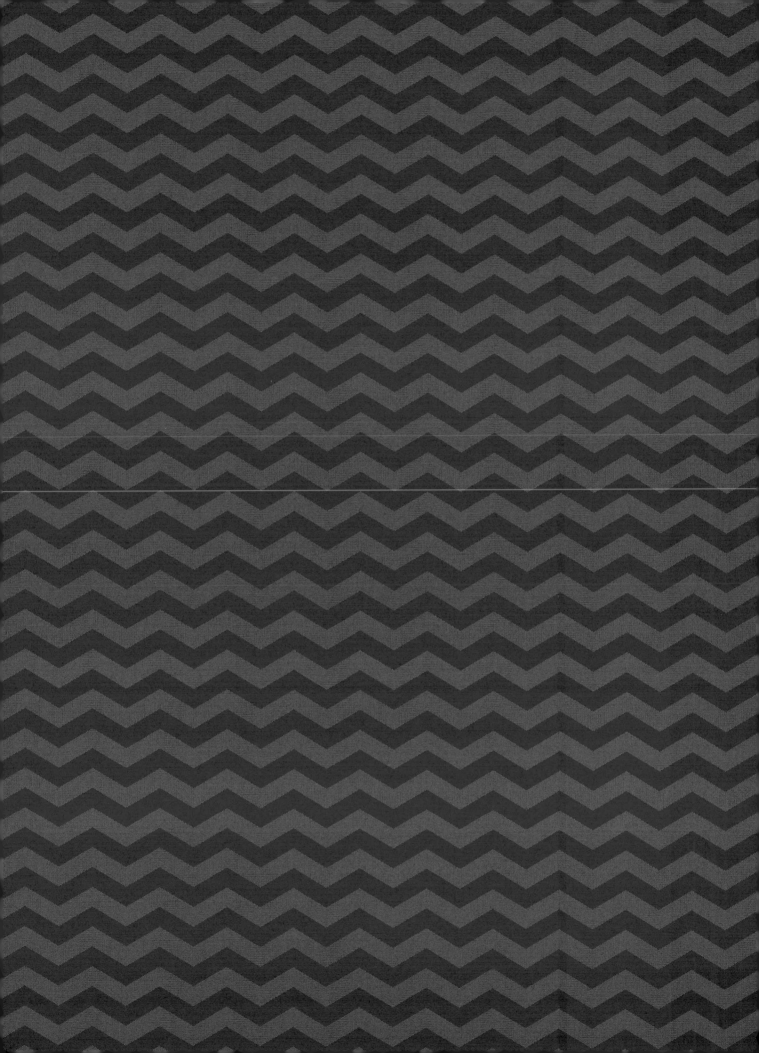

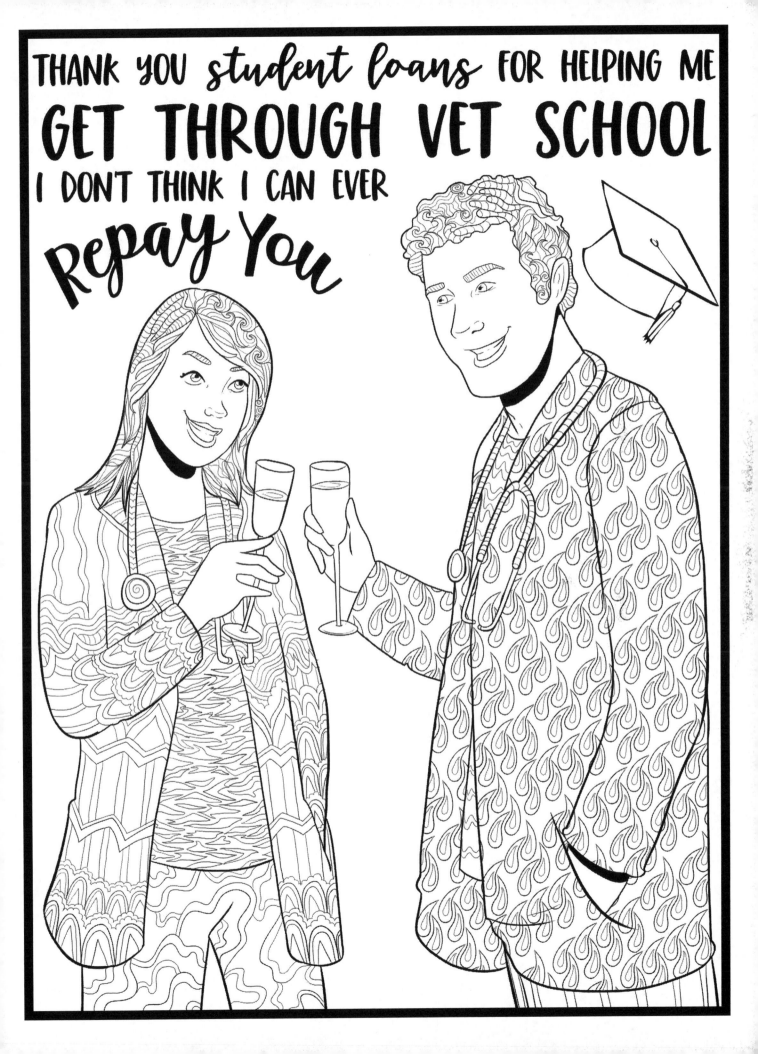

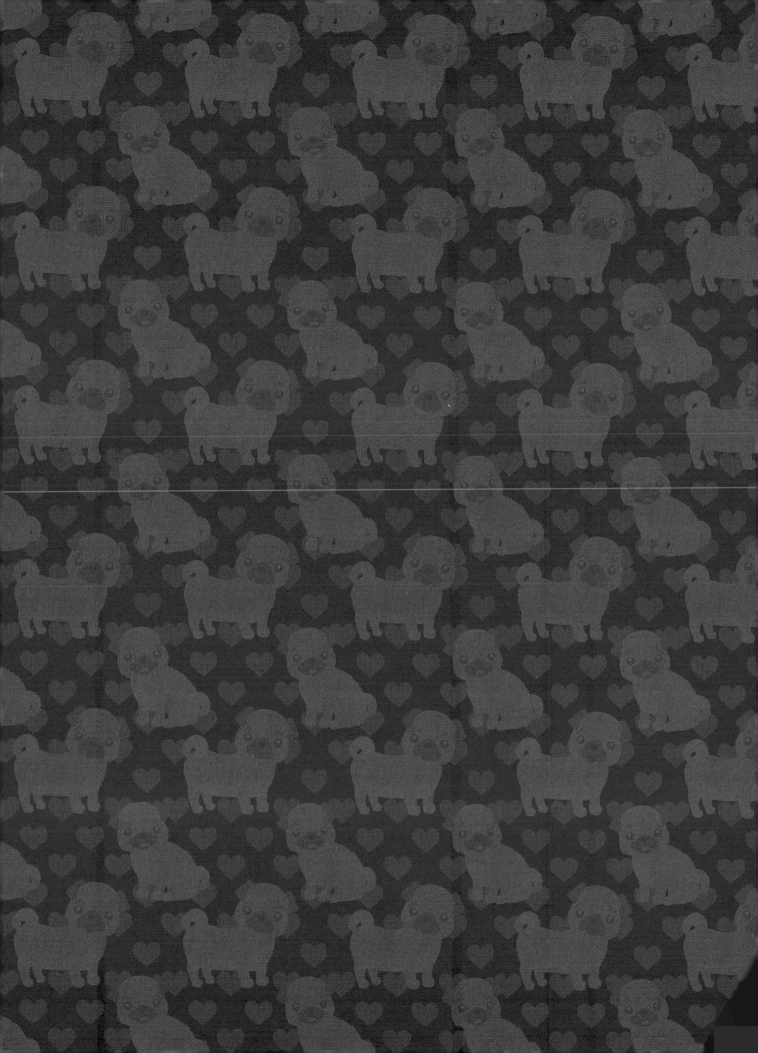

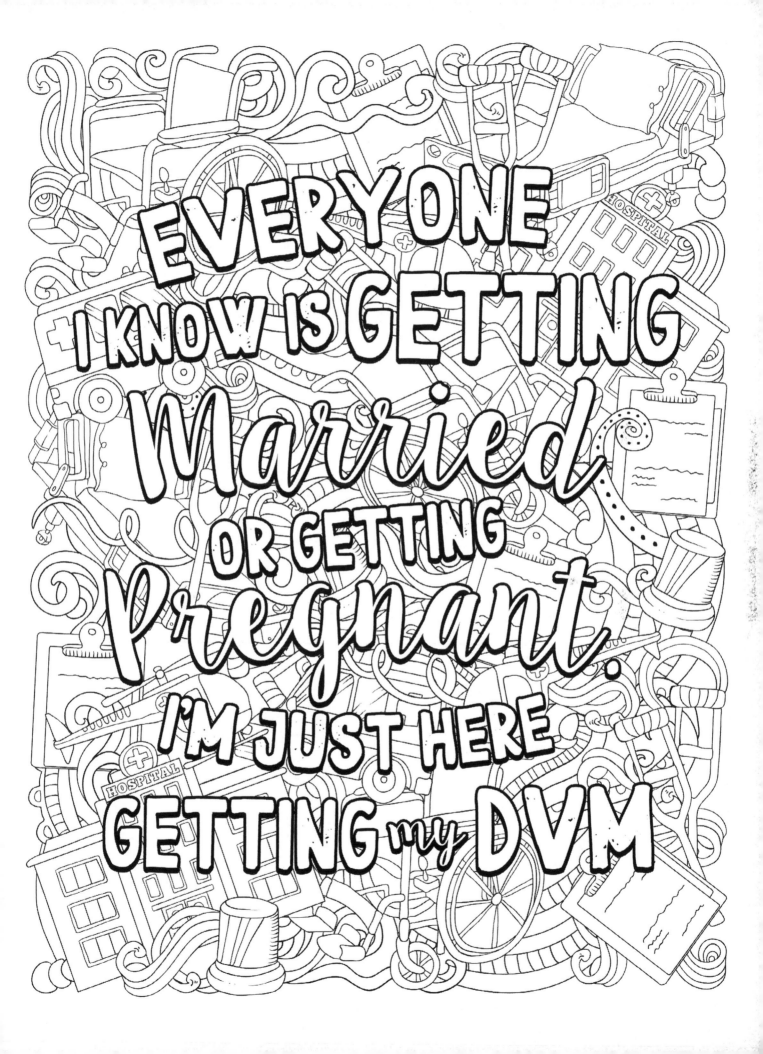

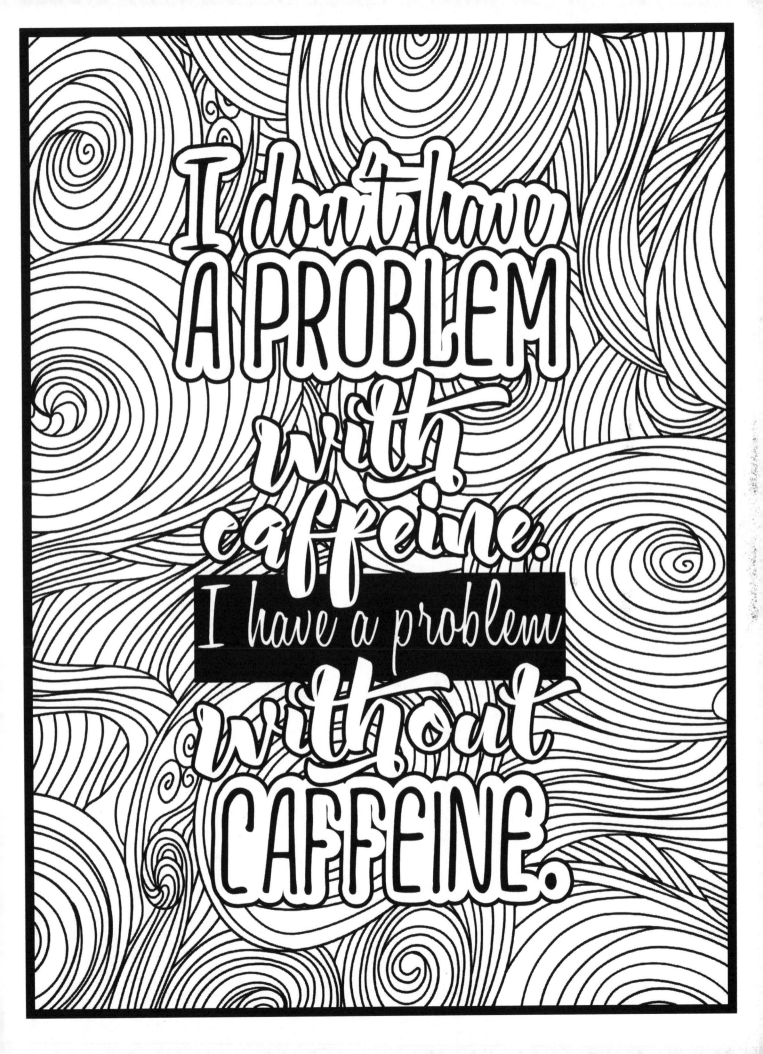

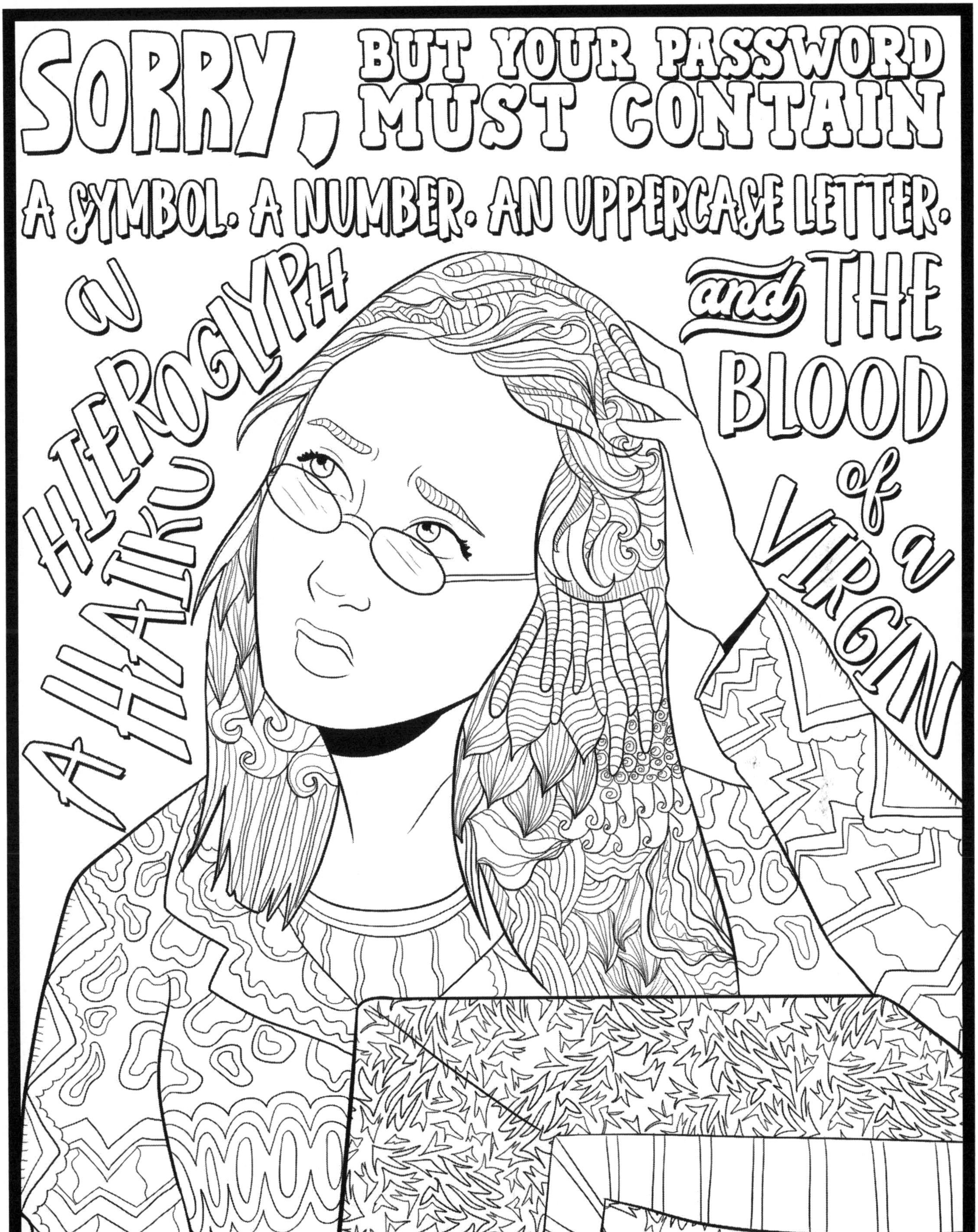
SORRY, BUT YOUR PASSWORD MUST CONTAIN
A SYMBOL. A NUMBER. AN UPPERCASE LETTER.
a HIEROGLYPH
A HAIKU
and THE BLOOD of a VIRGIN

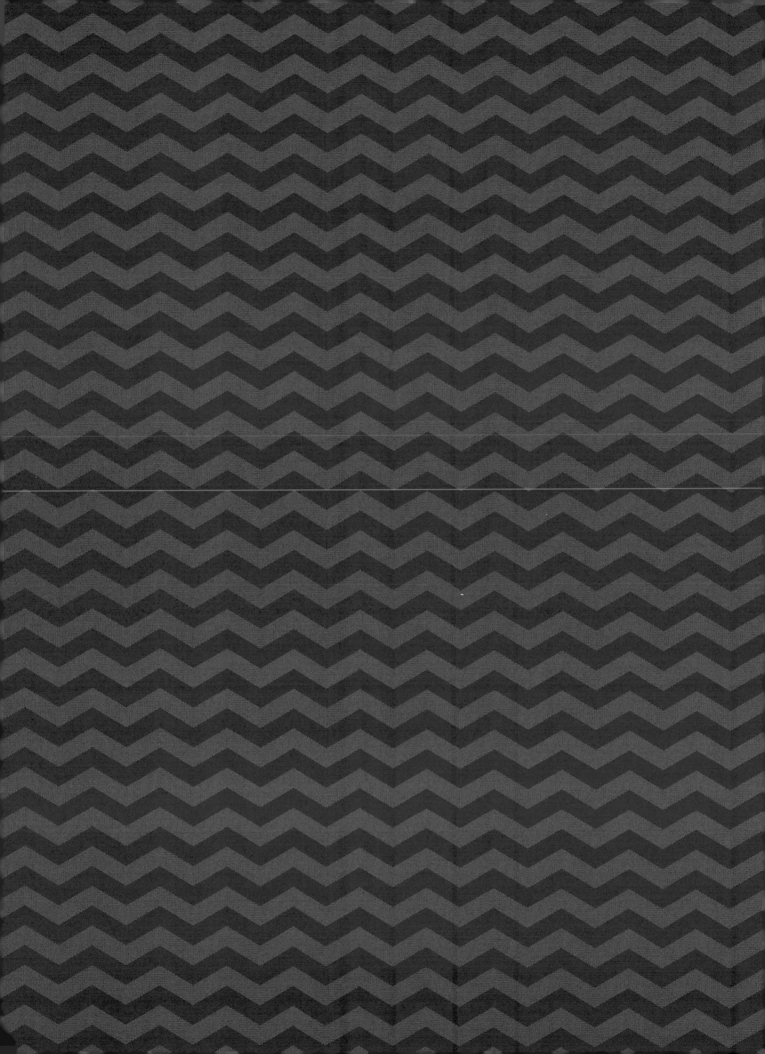

When U get A
Bladder
Infection

URINE
TROUBLE

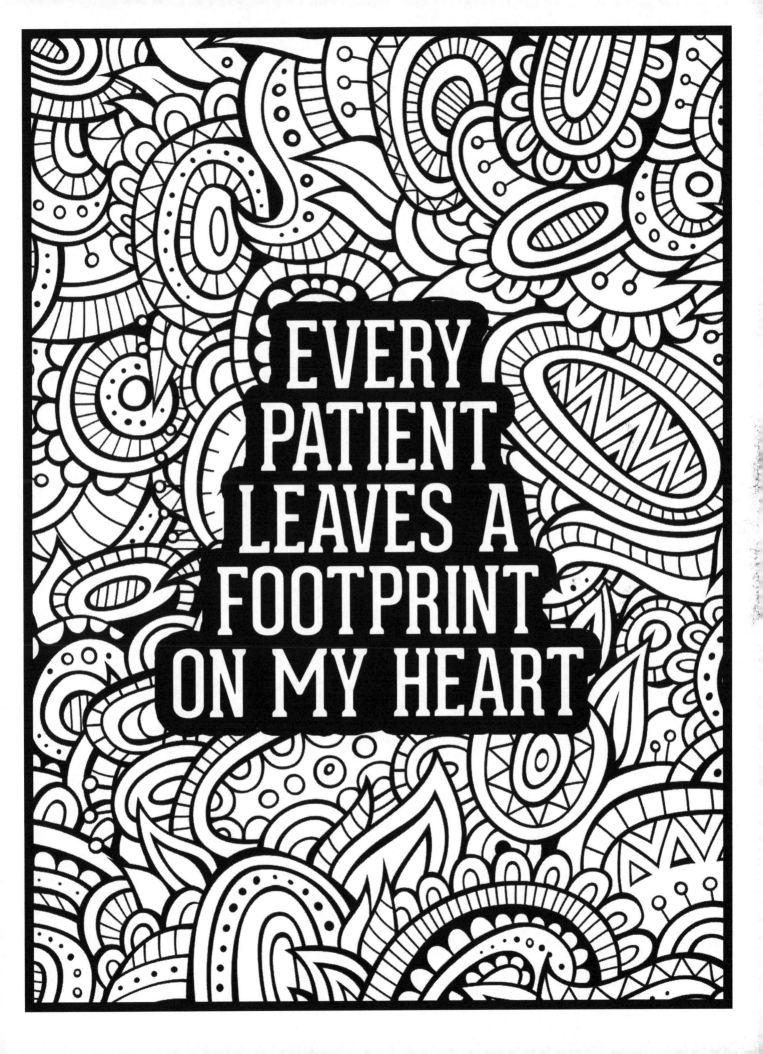

FREE DOWNLOAD

CODE BROWN does not MEAN SOMEONE brought CHOCOLATES

Never pass up an OPPORTUNITY to pee

BEHIND EVERY STABLE, WELL-ADJUSTED VET IS A PET OWNER WAITING TO CHANGE THAT BEFORE THE SHIFT is over

www.papeteriebleu.com/vetlife
YOUR DOWNLOAD CODE: VET3793

@papeteriebleu

f Papeterie Bleu

BE SURE TO FOLLOW US ON SOCIAL MEDIA FOR THE LATEST NEWS, SNEAK PEEKS, & GIVEAWAYS

[Instagram] @PapeterieBleu

[Facebook] Papeterie Bleu

[Twitter] @PapeterieBleu

ADD YOURSELF TO OUR MONTHLY NEWSLETTER FOR FREE DIGITAL DOWNLOADS AND DISCOUNT CODES

www.papeteriebleu.com/newsletter

CHECK OUT OUR OTHER BOOKS!

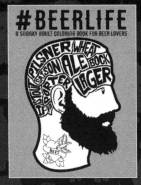

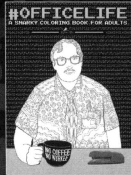

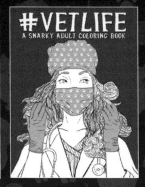

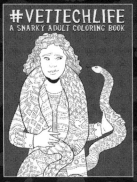

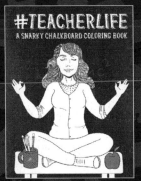

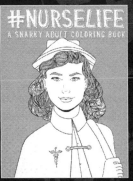

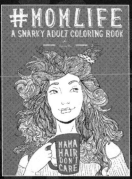

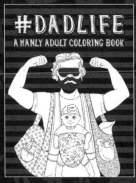

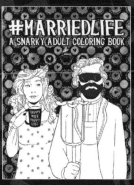

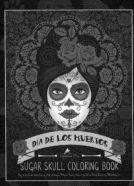

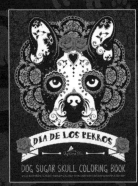

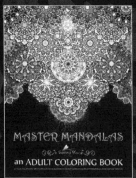

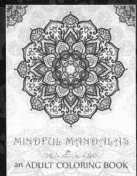

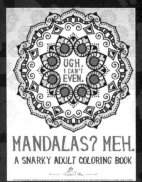

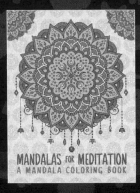

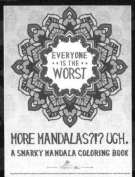

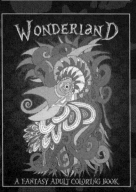

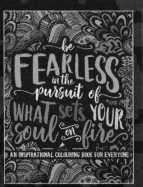

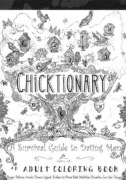

CHECK OUT OUR OTHER BOOKS!

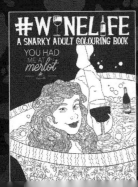

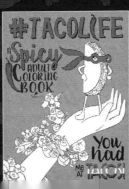

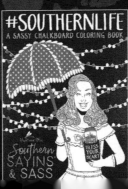

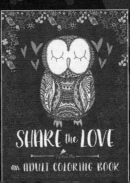

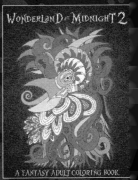

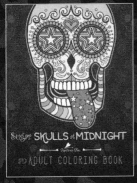

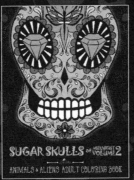

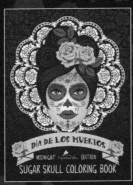

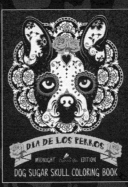

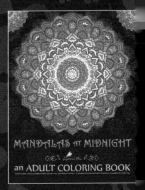

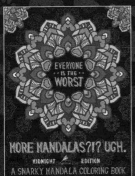

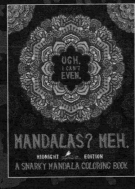

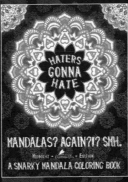

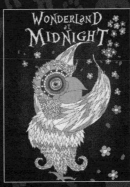

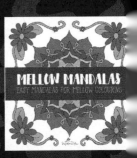

CHECK OUT OUR OTHER BOOKS!

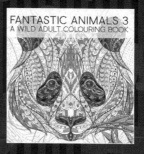

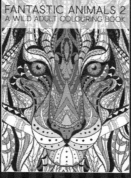

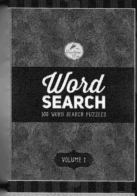

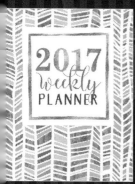

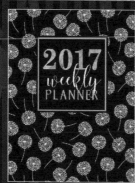

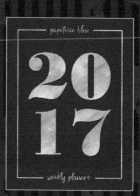

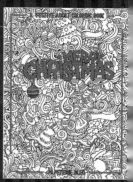

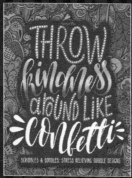

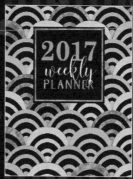

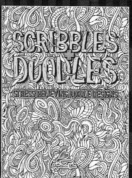

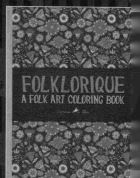

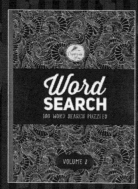

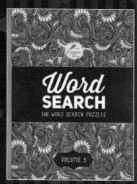

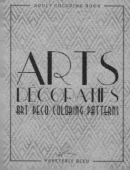

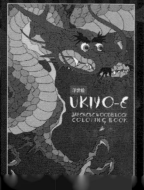

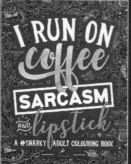

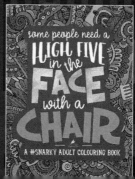

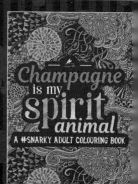

Made in the USA
San Bernardino, CA
09 July 2019